We would like to extend our deepest gratitude to the following sponsors whose generosity, compassion, and unwavering support played a significant role in making *The Ribbon* a success.

We are grateful for your willingness to stand beside us and help spread a message of hope, resilience, and awareness to those children and families who have faced a medical diagnosis.

Thank you for believing in the message, supporting the mission and helping us remind others that they are never alone.

with Threads of Gratitude

Dr. Greg and Chris Hansen

The Henderson Family

Dr. Julie Statz and Family

The Stutts Family

Dr. Tyler Rogers and Family

The Wood Family

Kathy Hansen

The Mahoney Family

The Hinkeldey and Family

The Quann Family

Erin Smith and Family

The Fisher Family

Jessica and Family

Dedicated to Ray, James, and the countless children whose strength reveals the true meaning of resilience.

In Memoriam of Hazel, whose light will always guide and shine upon her sisters and parents.

Published by 30 Press, LLC.
Written by Beth Seidl.
Cover Design, Illustrations, and Interior design by Hannah Roser.
Edited by Ashley Franz Holzmann.
Interior fonts are Arimo licensed under the Open Font License.
First edition first printed in 2026.
ISBN 978-1-962330-03-9
www.30press.com

The Ribbon

Written by: Beth Seidl

Illustrated by: Hannah Roser

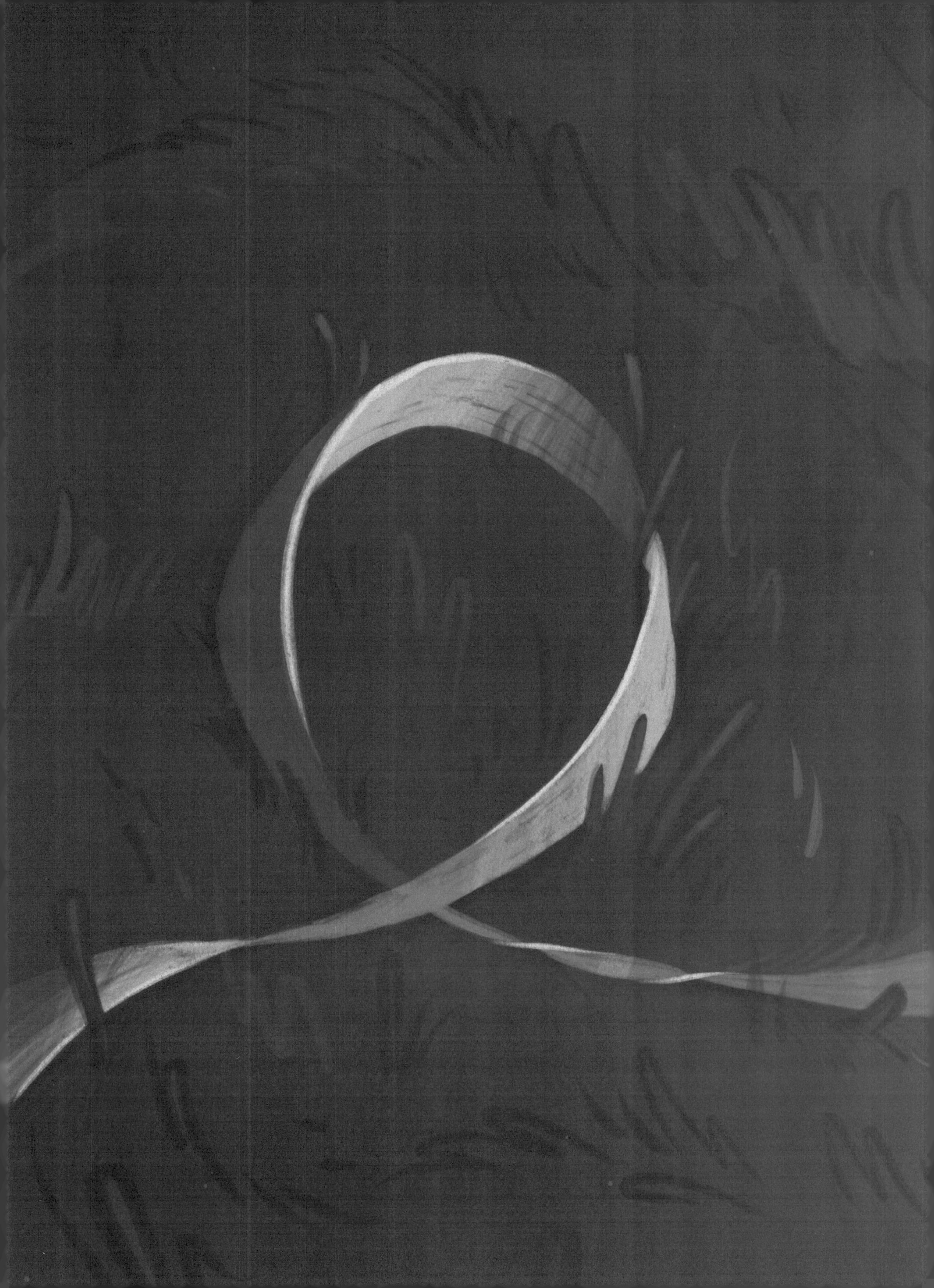

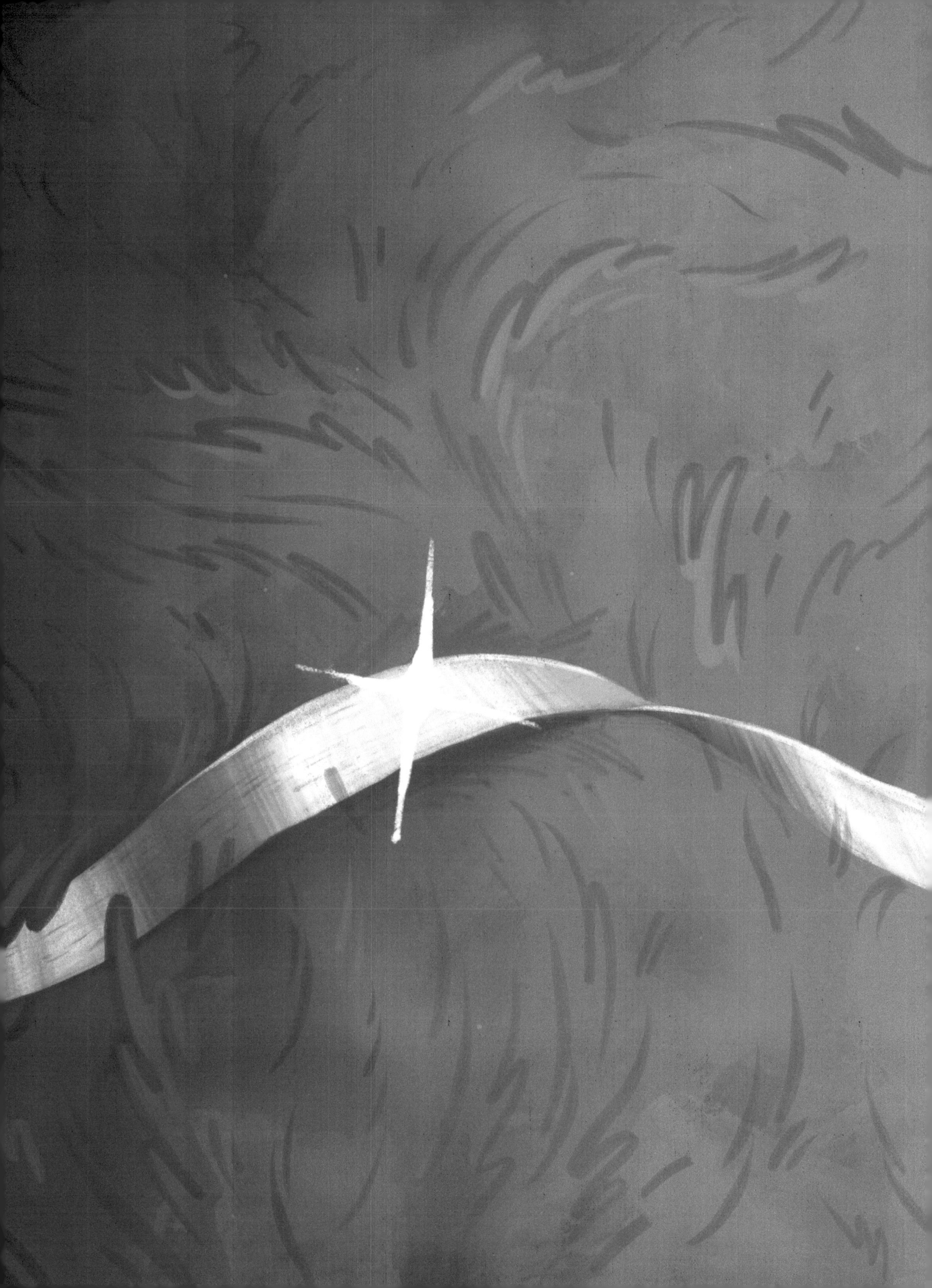

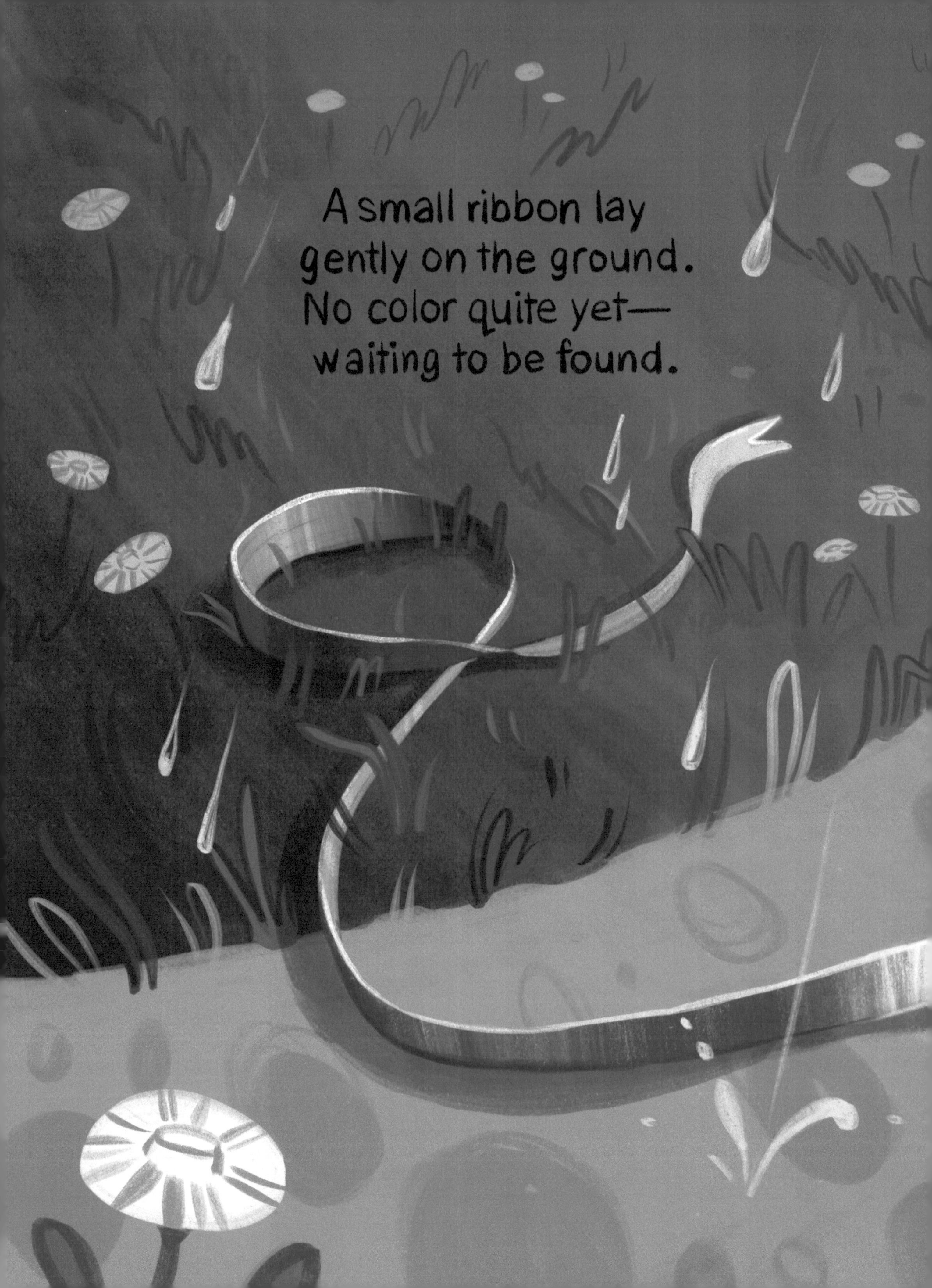

A small ribbon lay
gently on the ground.
No color quite yet—
waiting to be found.

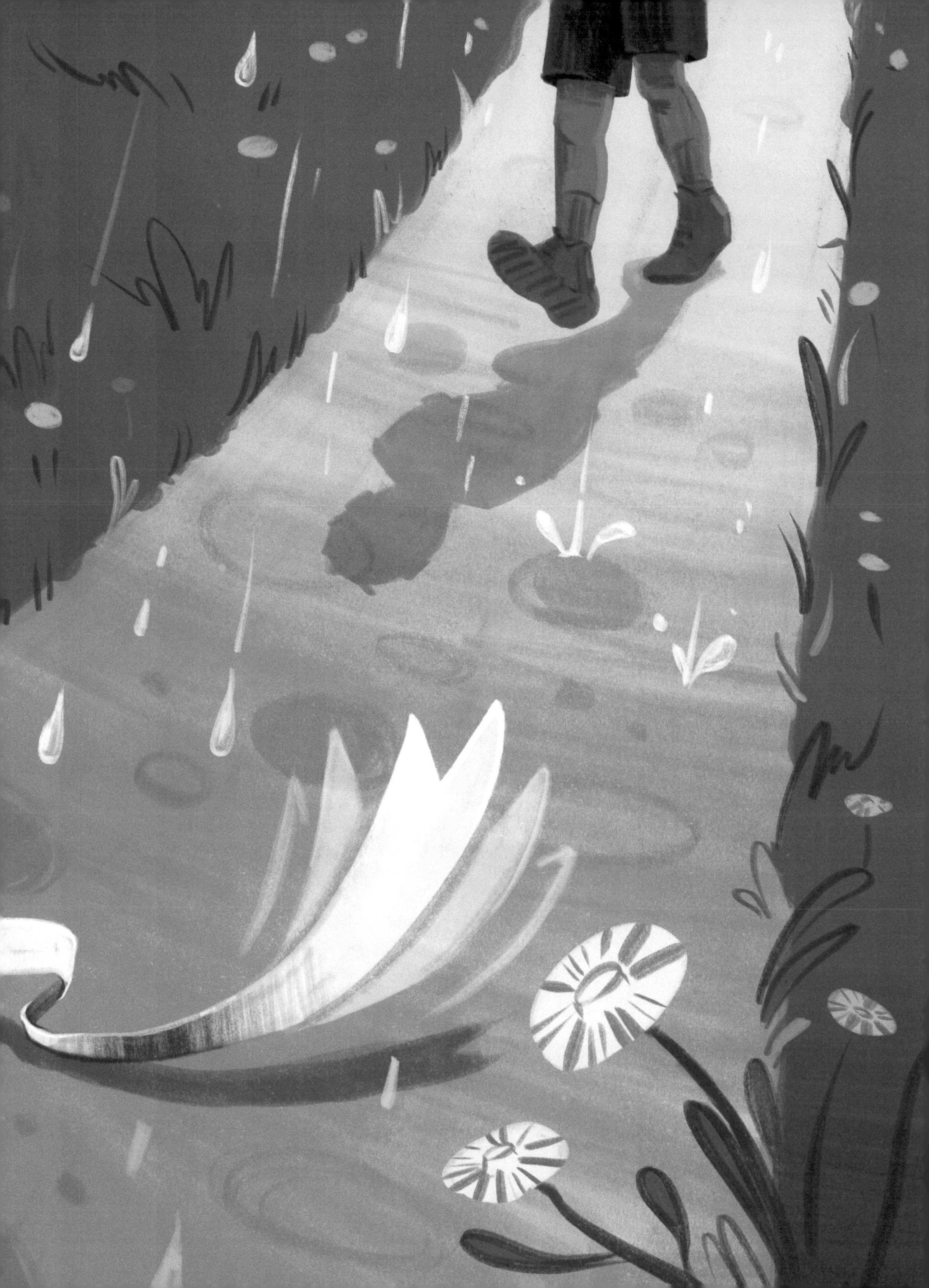

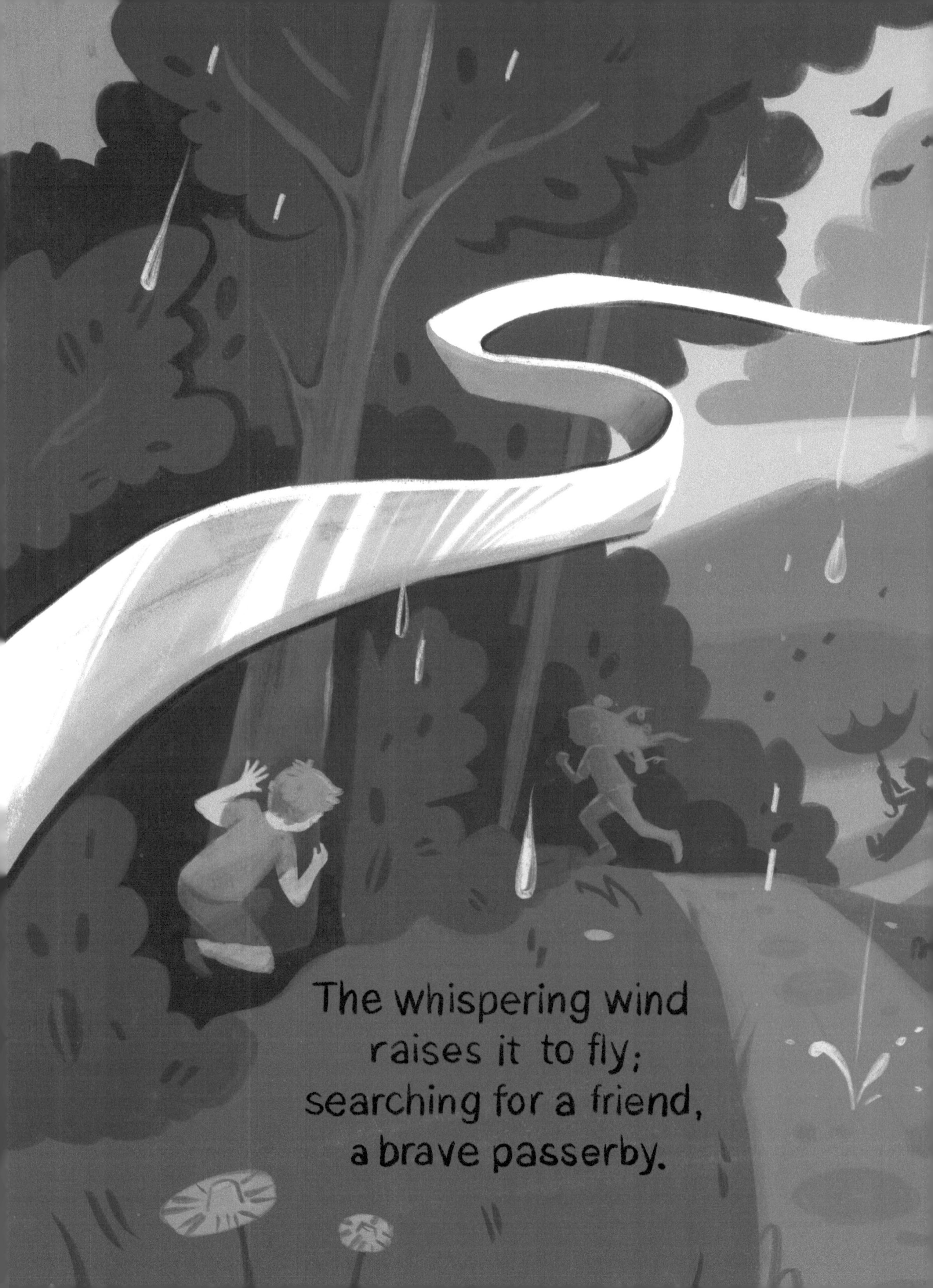

The whispering wind
raises it to fly;
searching for a friend,
a brave passerby.

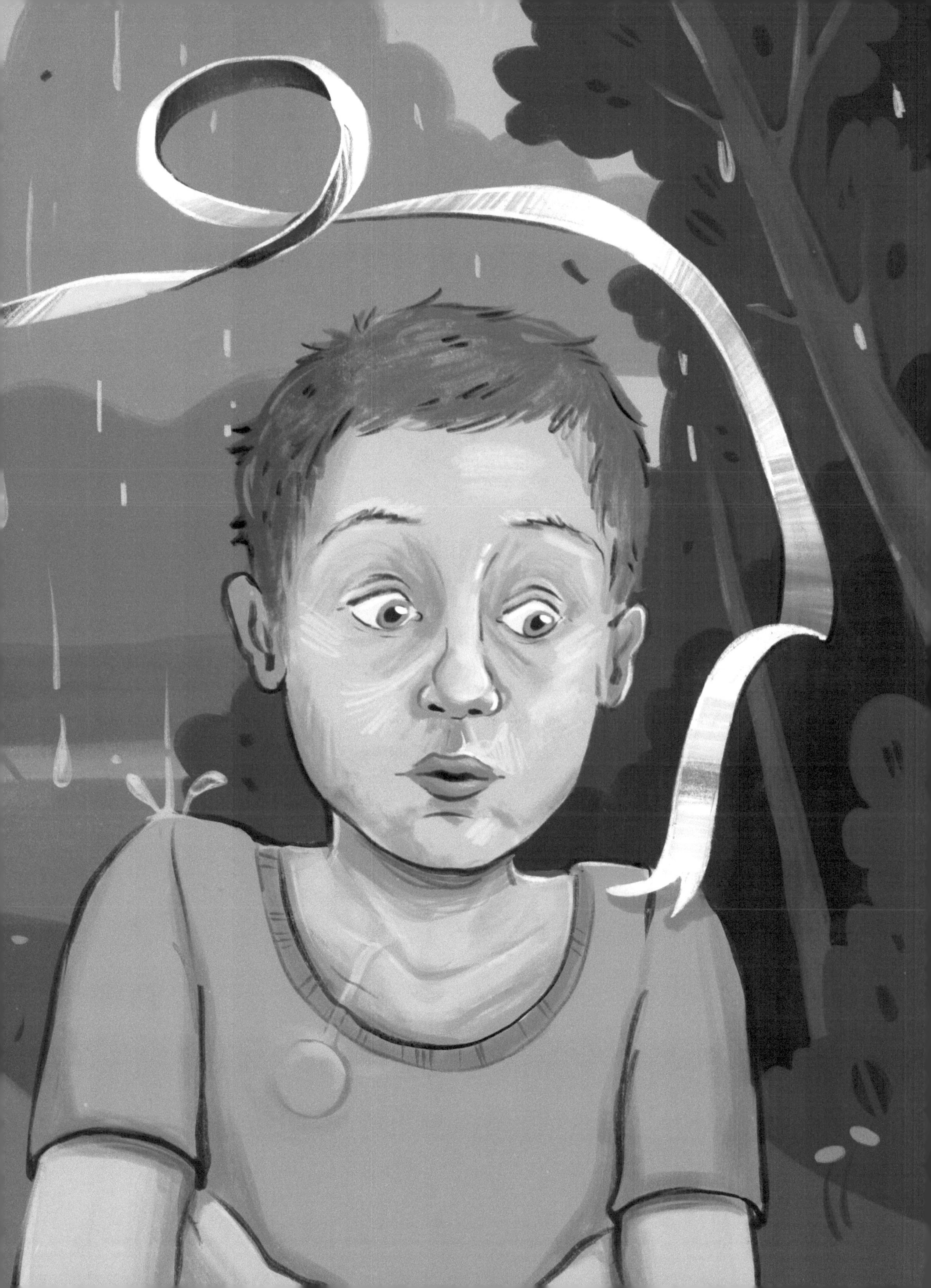

The child feels seen,
The ribbon in sight.

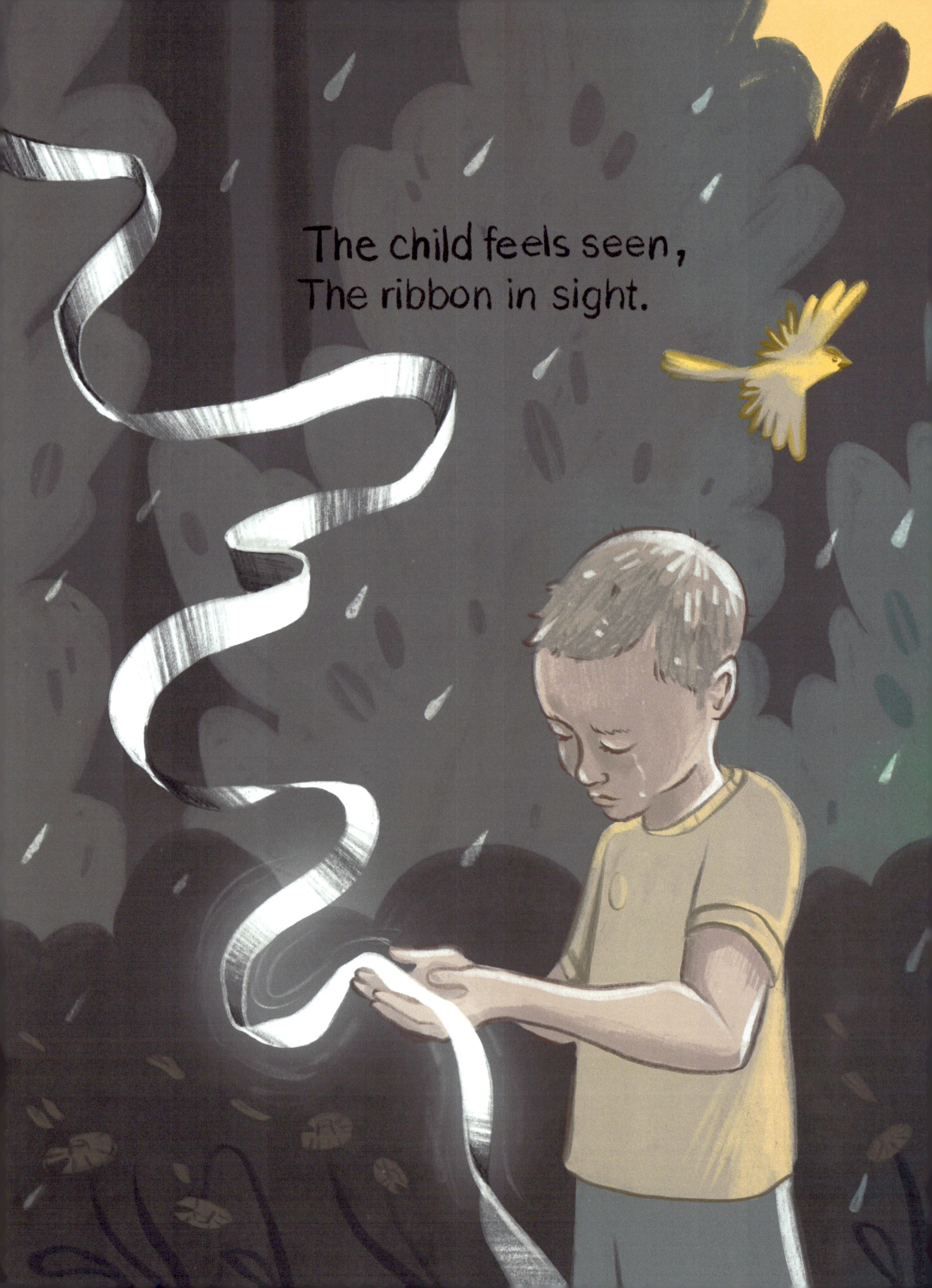

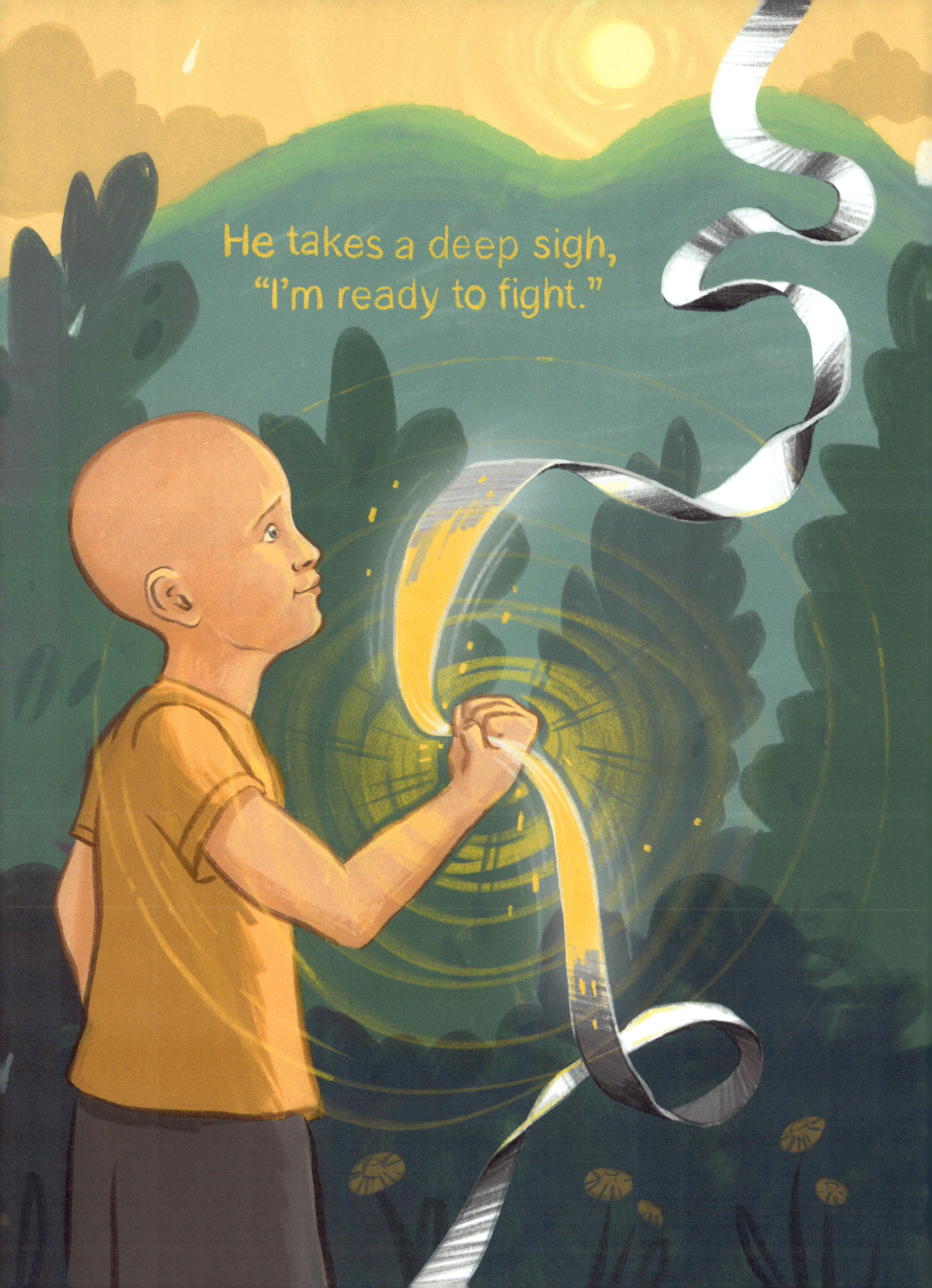

He takes a deep sigh,
"I'm ready to fight."

Single loop in hand,
the thread turns to gold.
Journeys through treatments
for all those so bold.

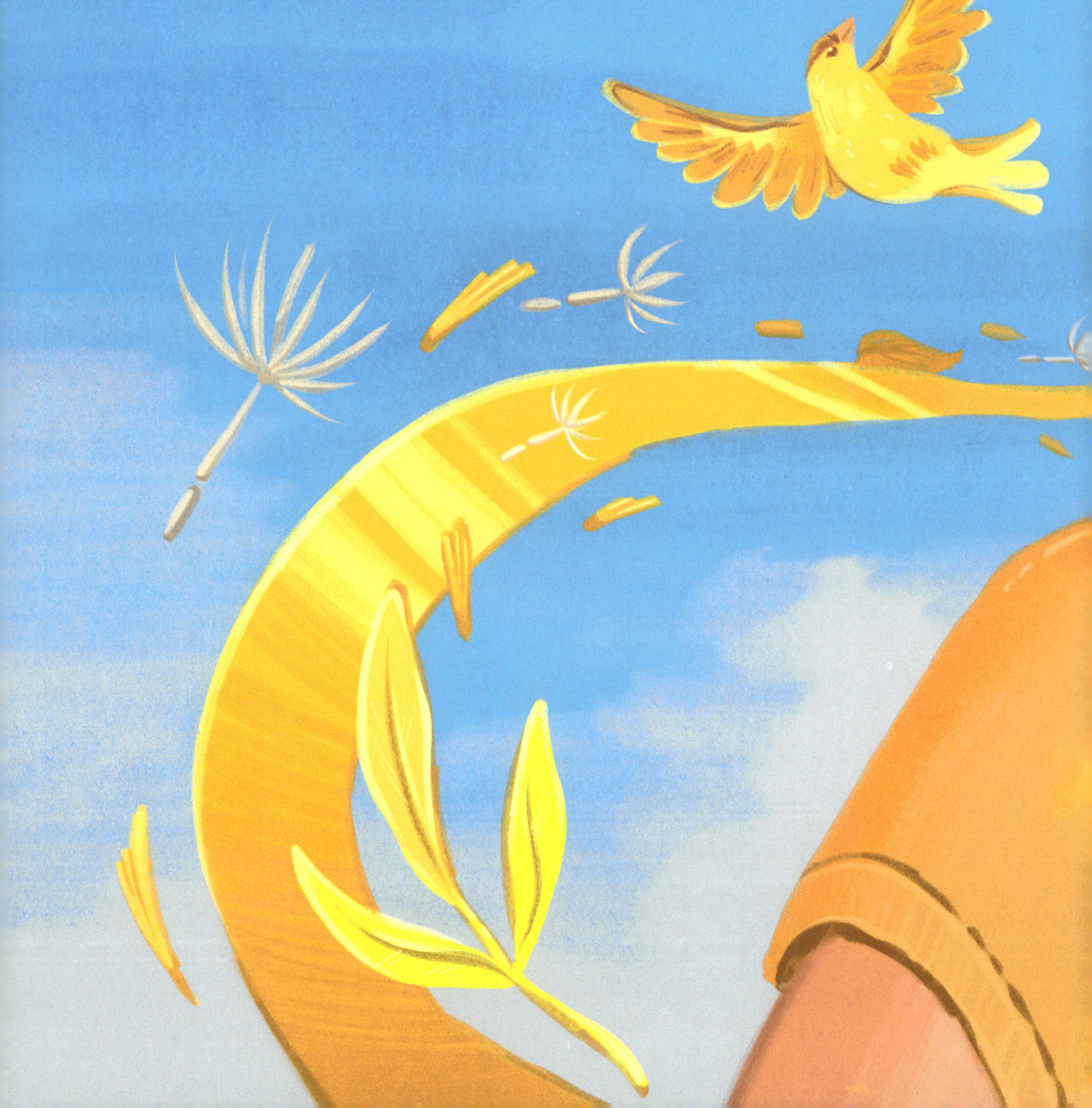

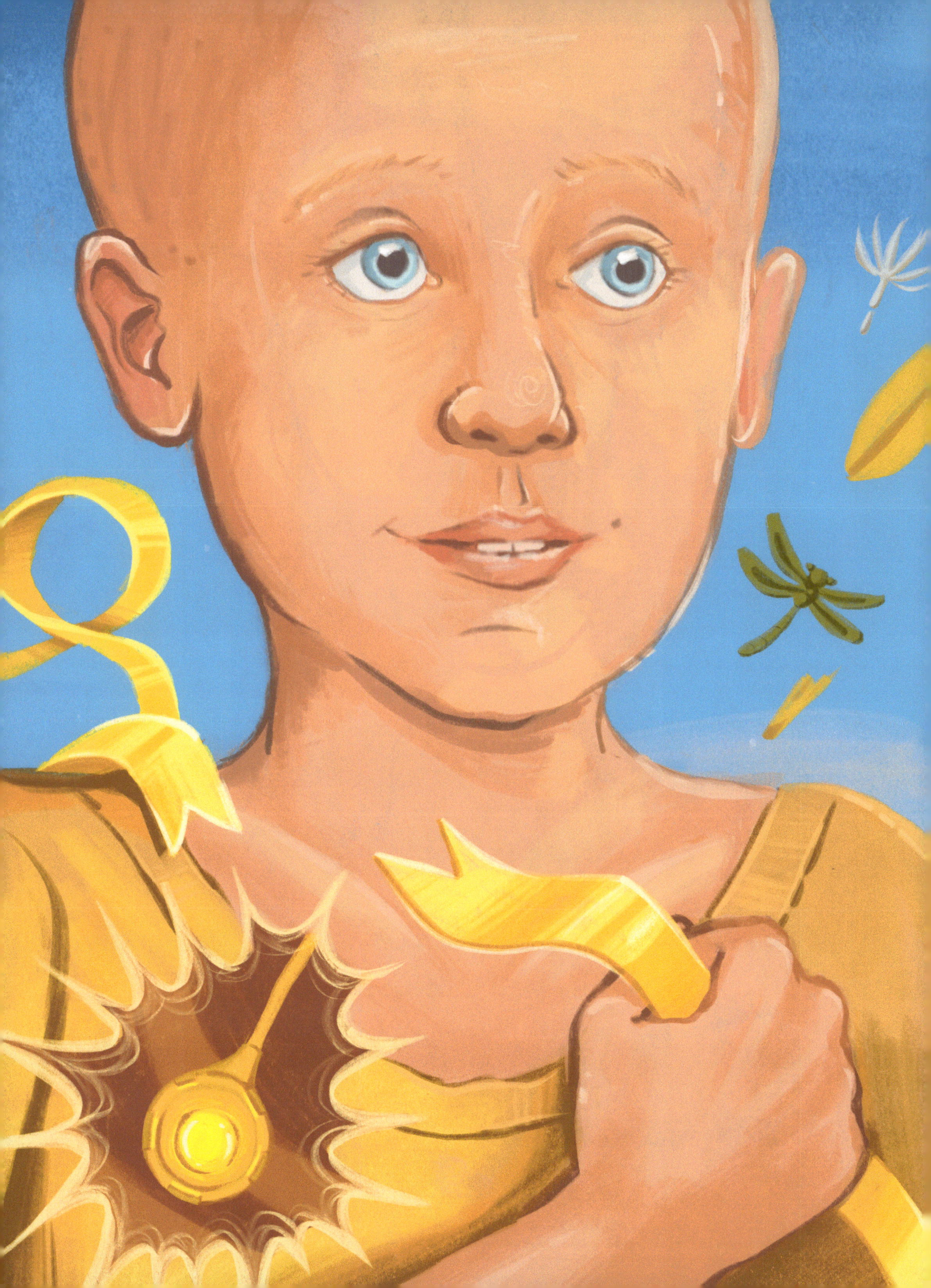

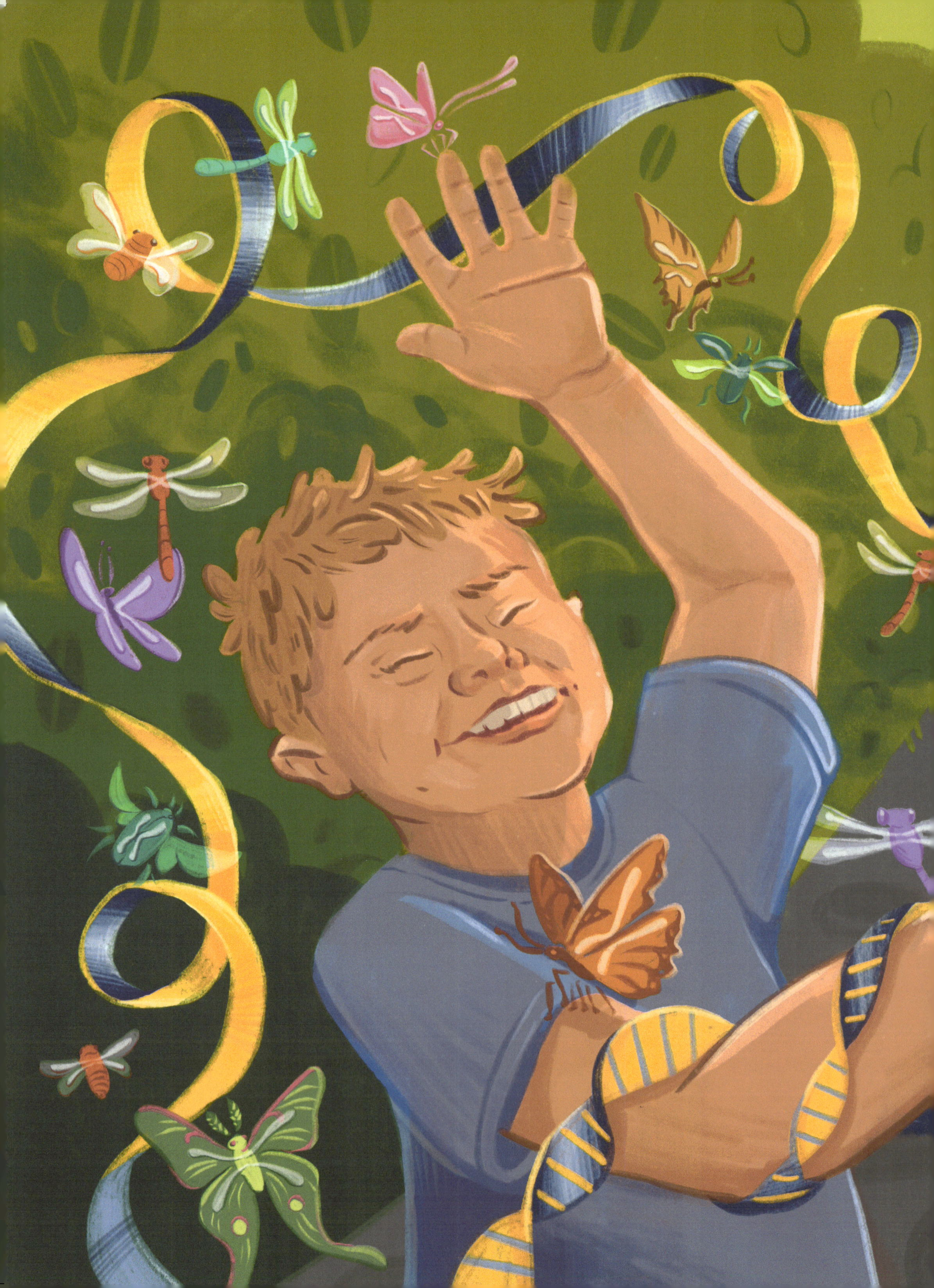

One curve not enough,
the ribbon seeks more.
Joy for one "extra",
this child to adore.

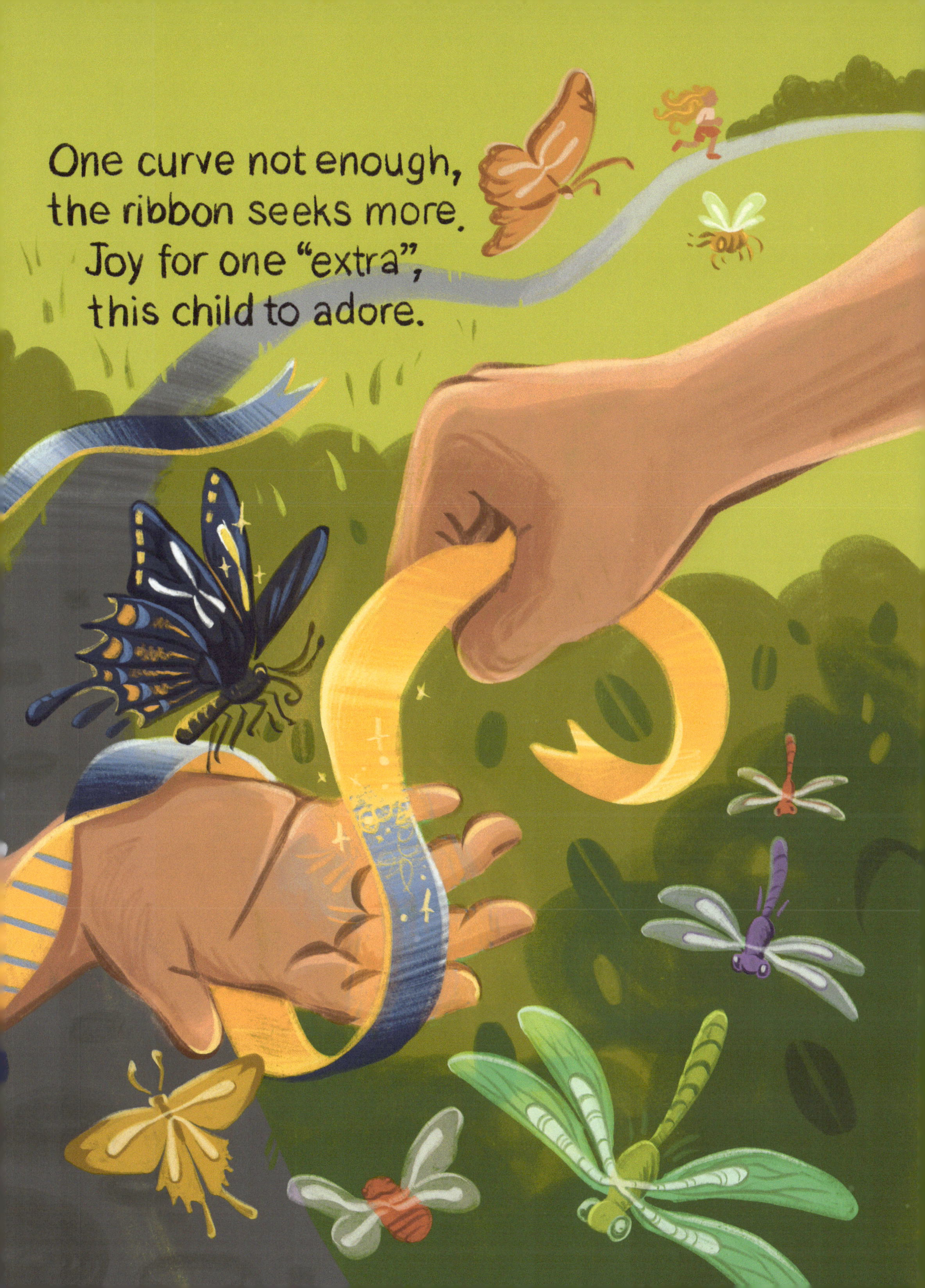

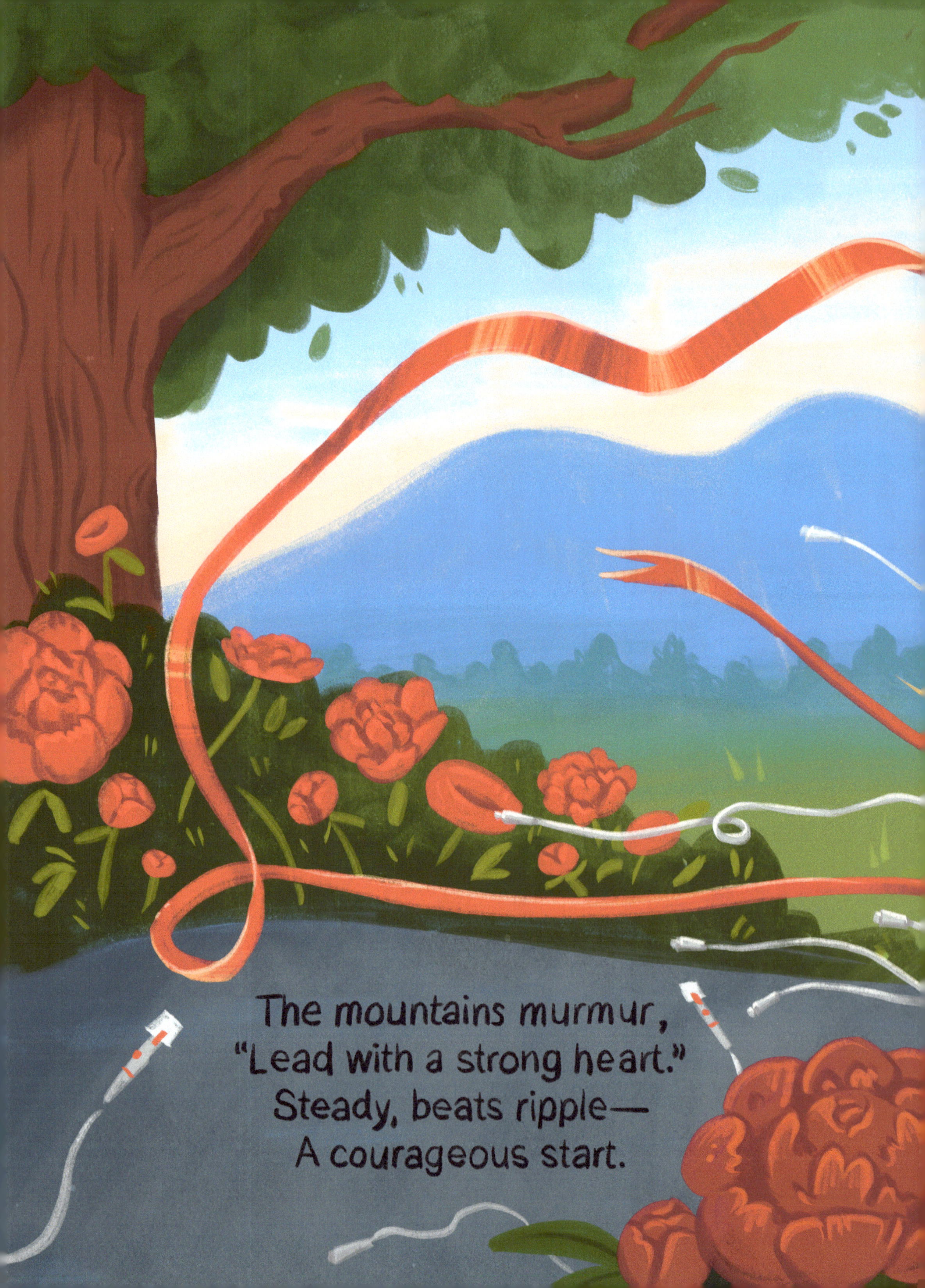

The mountains murmur,
"Lead with a strong heart."
Steady, beats ripple—
A courageous start.

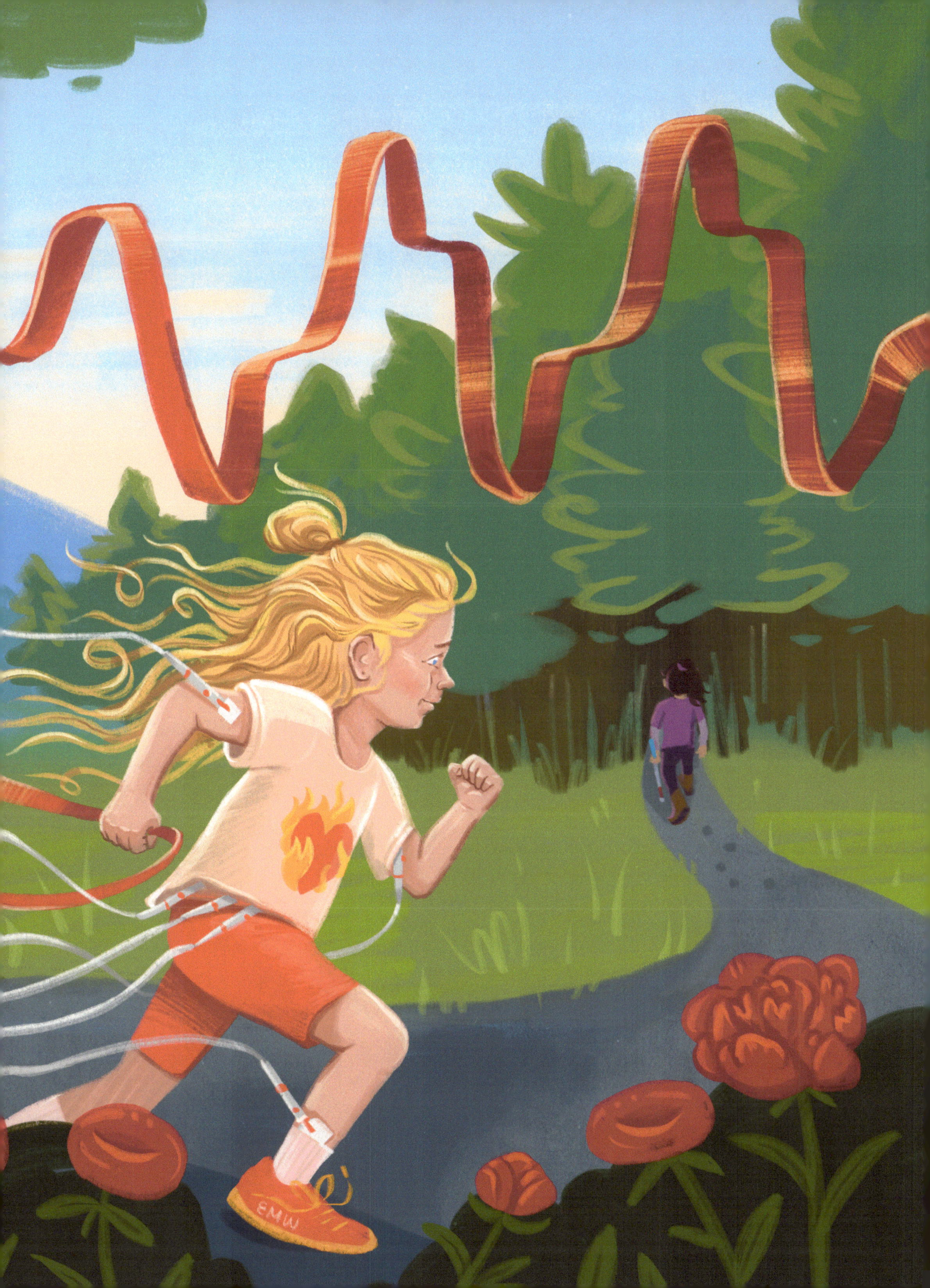
EMW

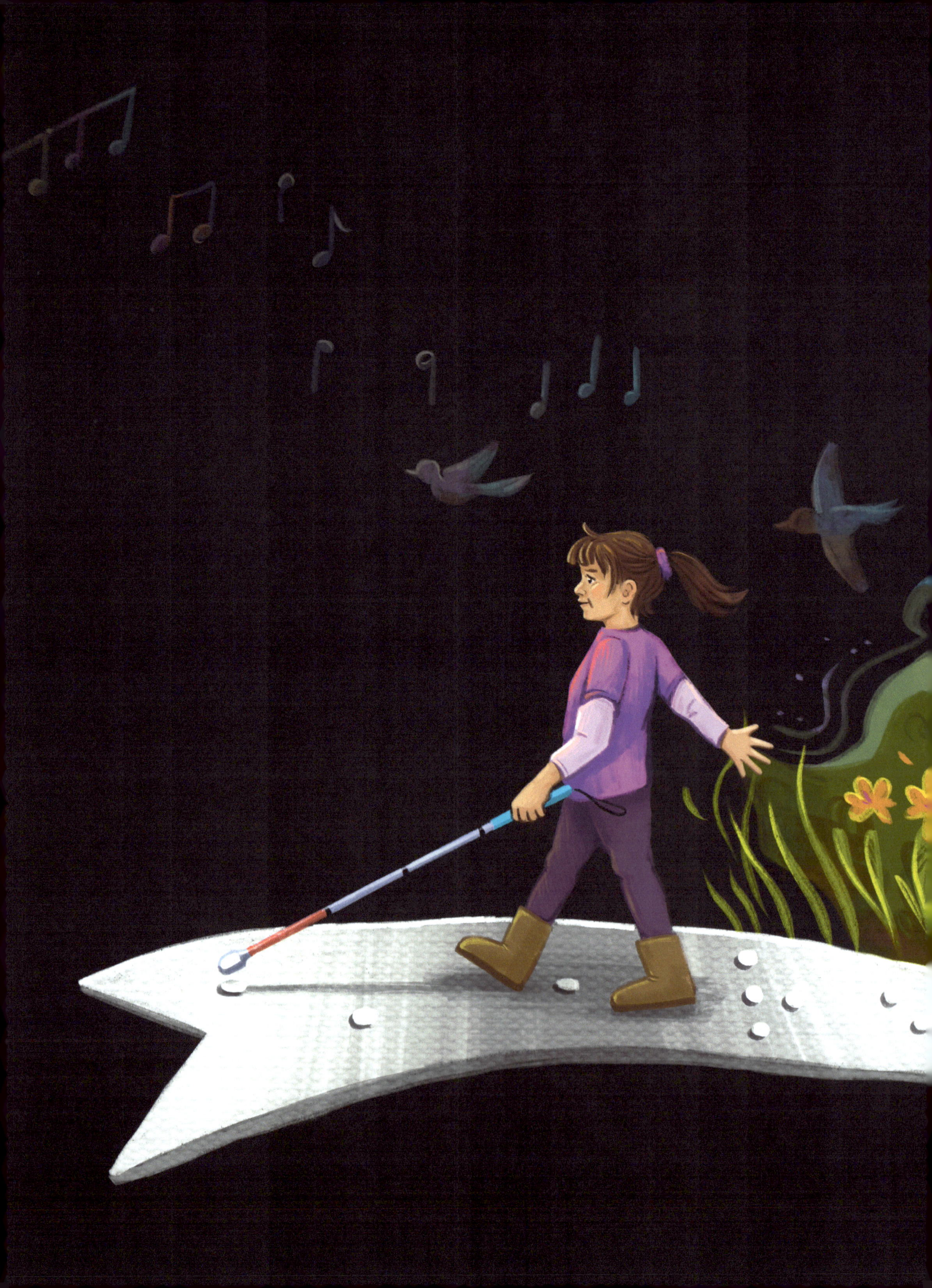

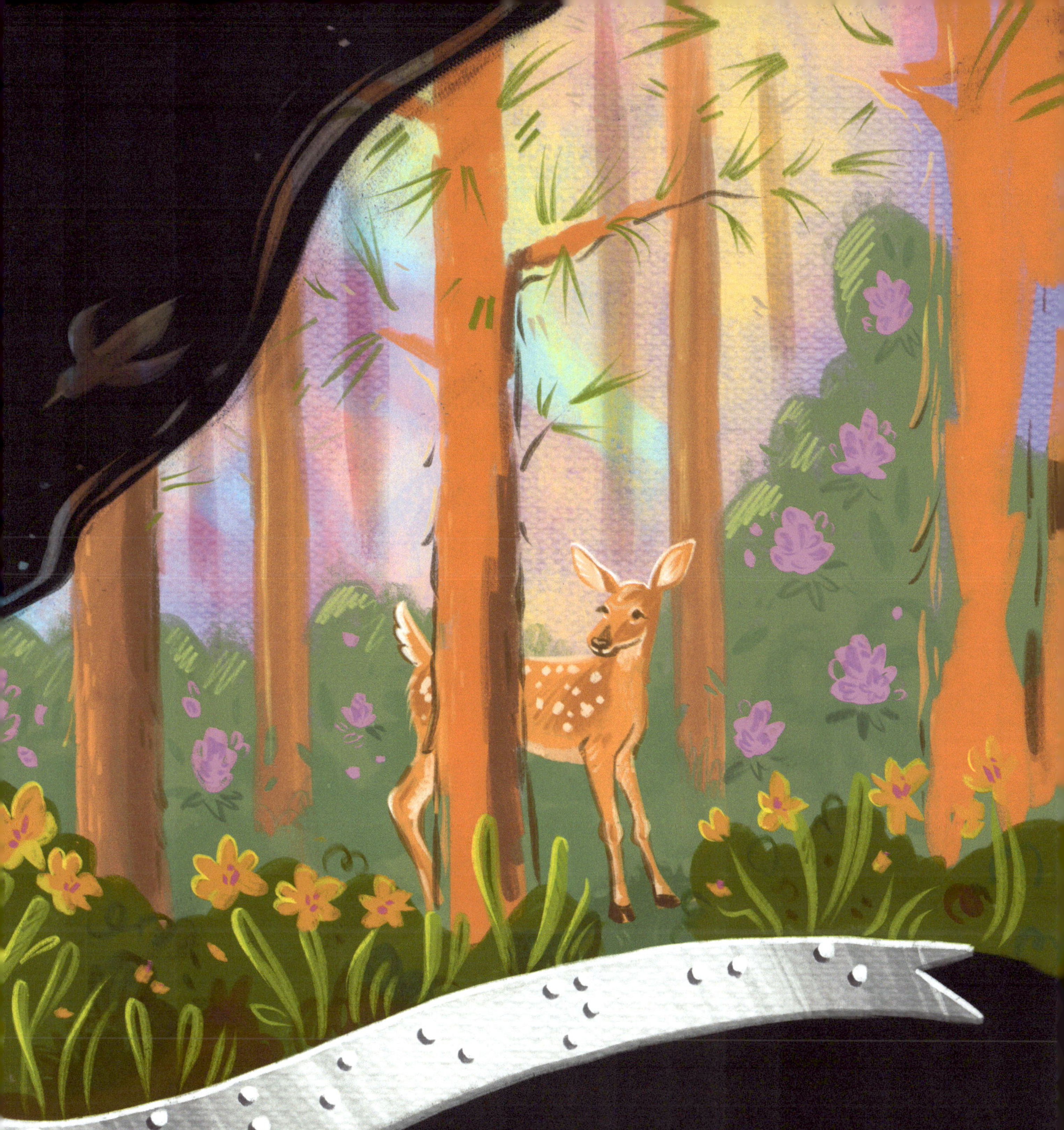

A canvas awaits—
you are its keeper.
For what you can't see,
feels ever deeper.

The ribbon, a symbol;
of silence so loud.
It's spoken through hands;
without a sound.

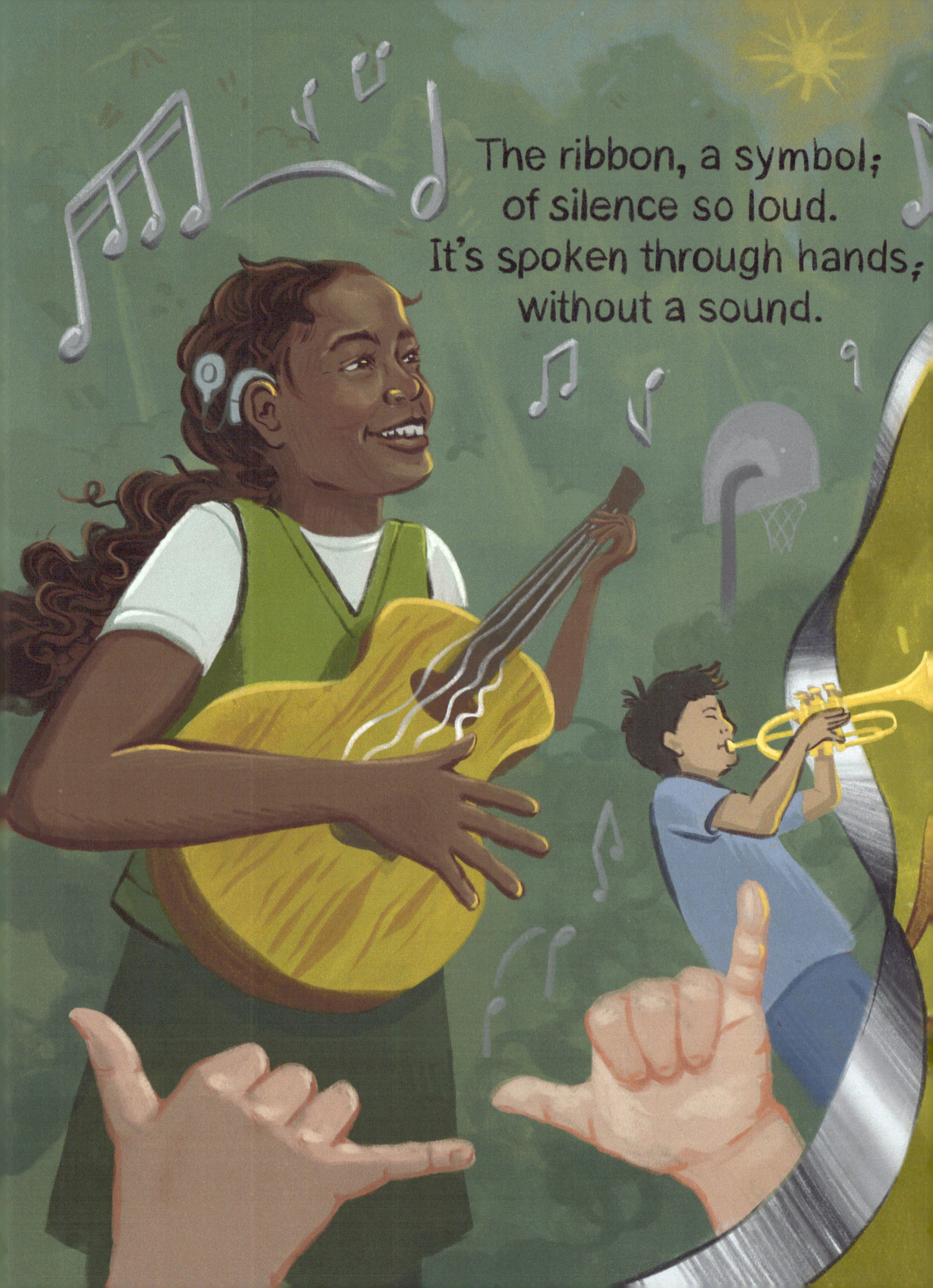

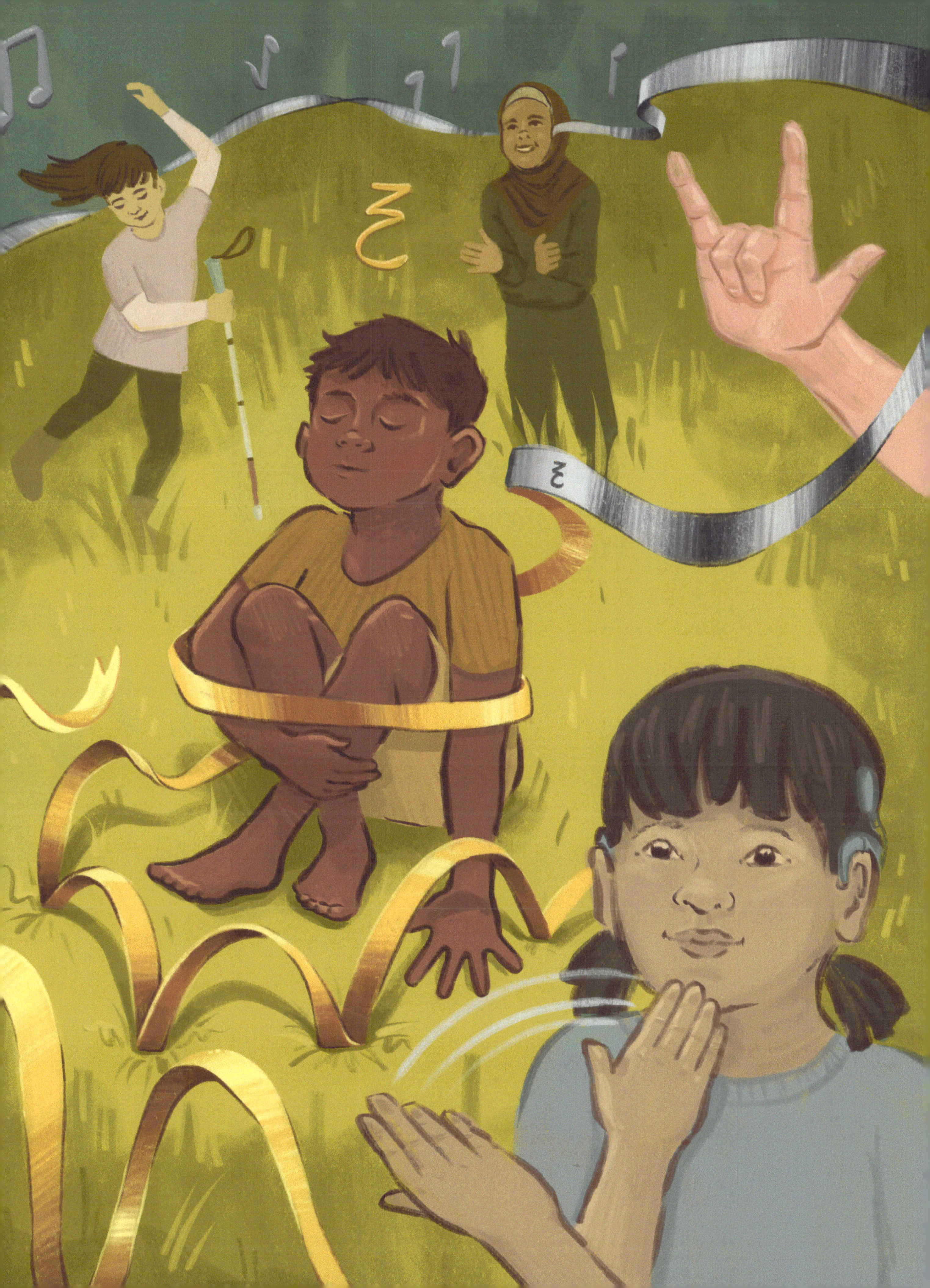
ع
ع

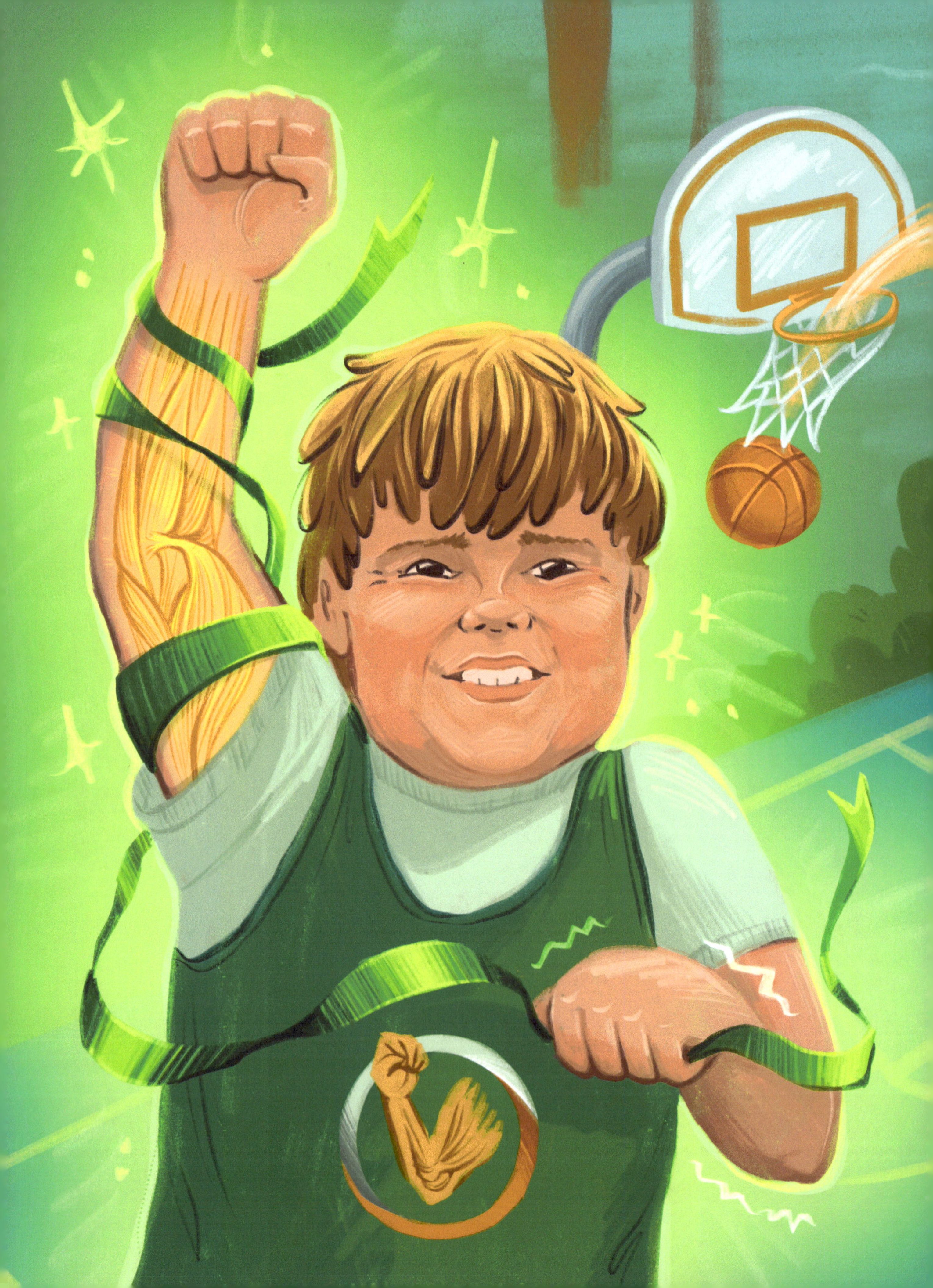

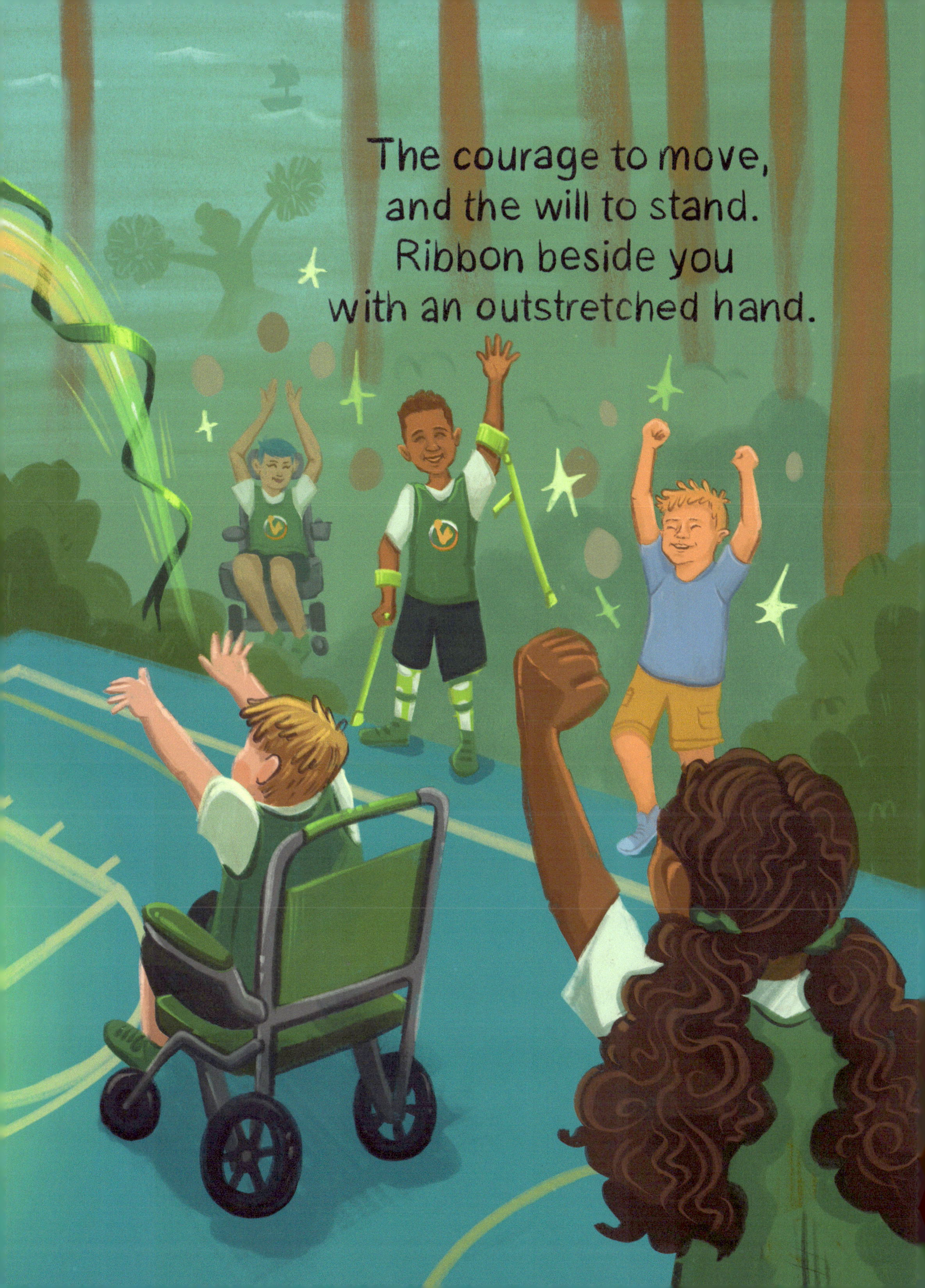

The courage to move,
and the will to stand.
Ribbon beside you
with an outstretched hand.

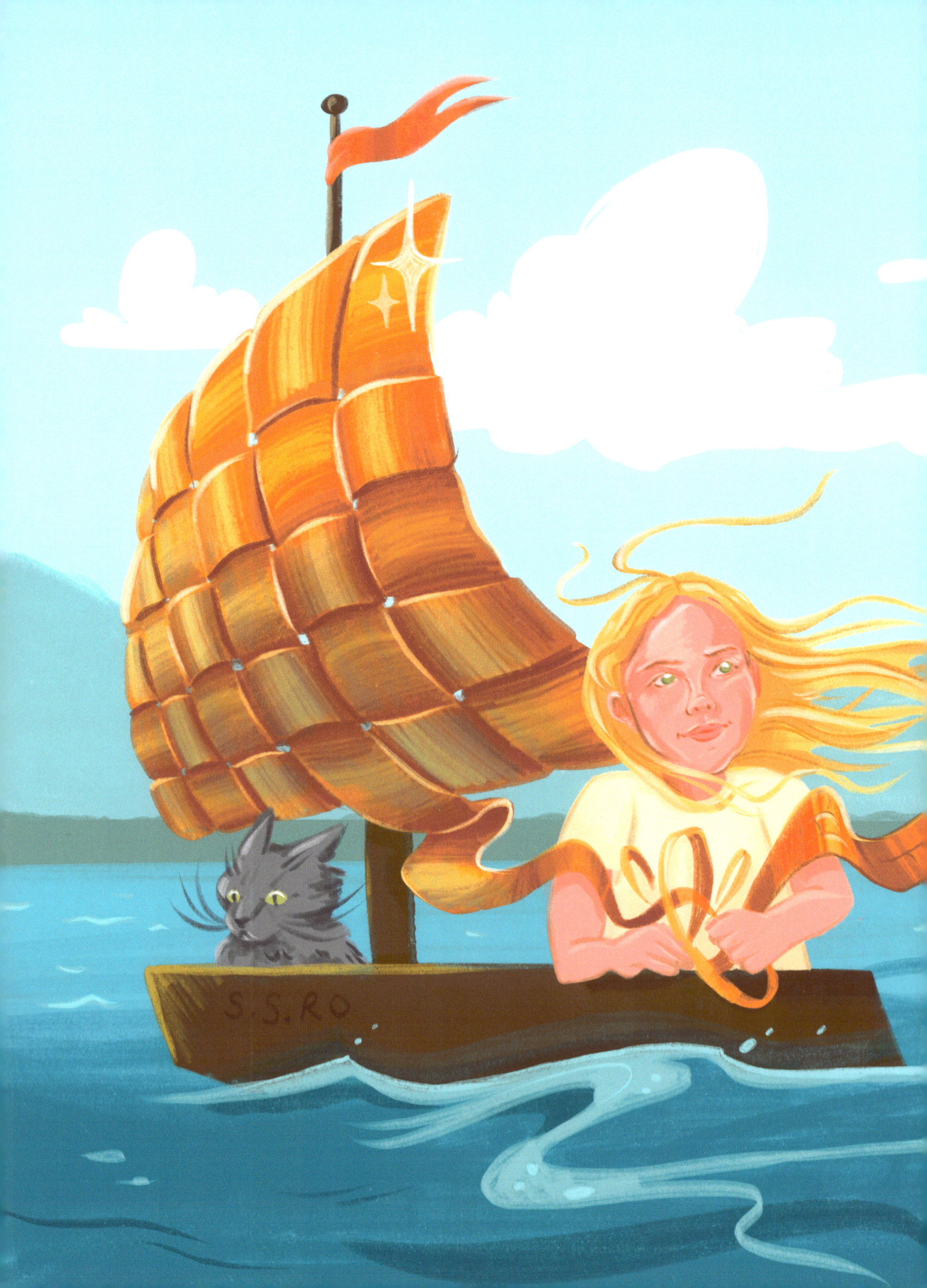
S.S.RO

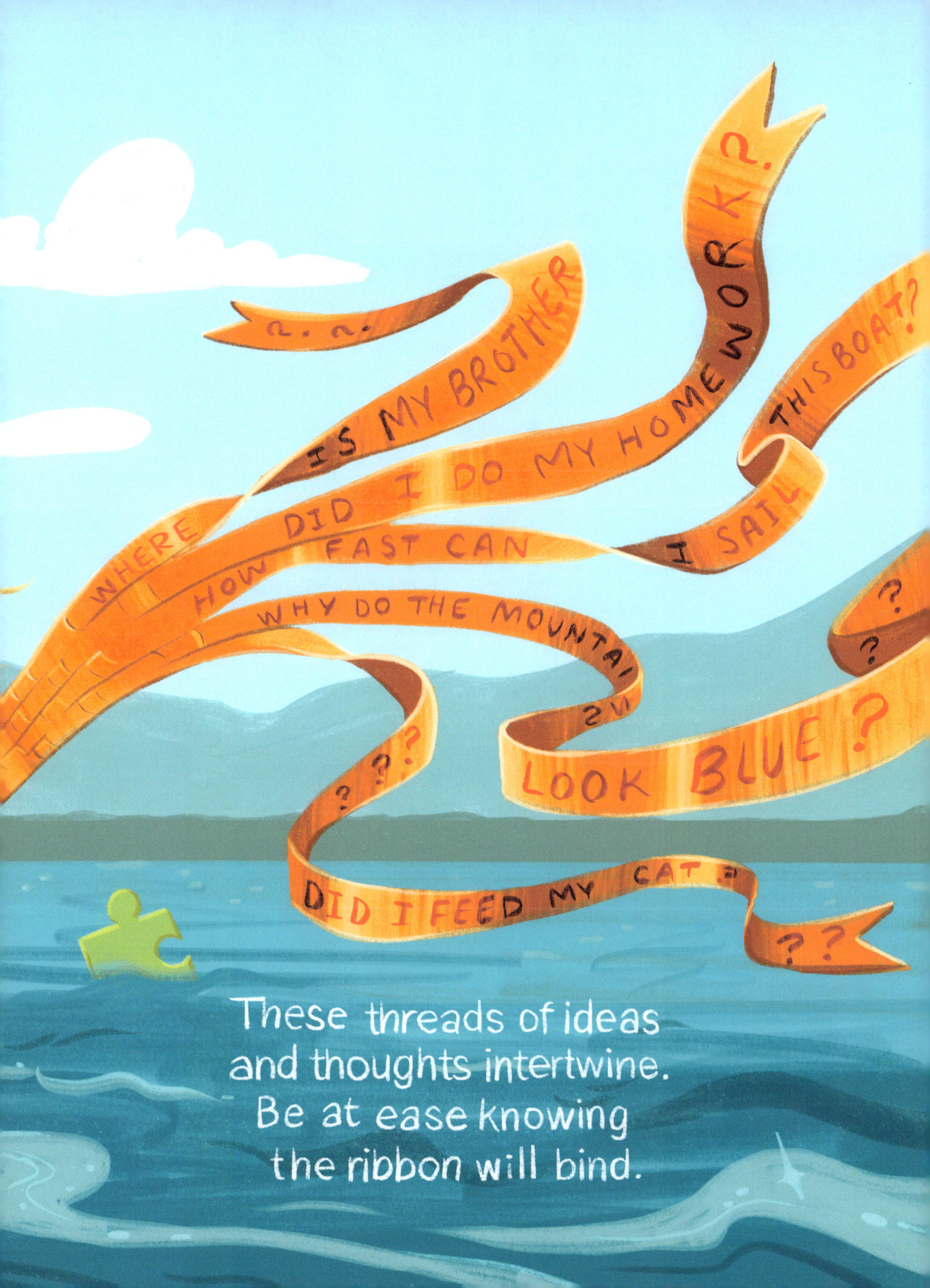
WHERE IS MY BROTHER ??
HOW DID I DO MY HOMEWORK?
HOW FAST CAN I SAIL THIS BOAT?
WHY DO THE MOUNTAINS LOOK BLUE ???
DID I FEED MY CAT ???

These threads of ideas
and thoughts intertwine.
Be at ease knowing
the ribbon will bind.

Decipher each word,
a puzzle to solve.
A moment of doubt,
but meaning evolves.

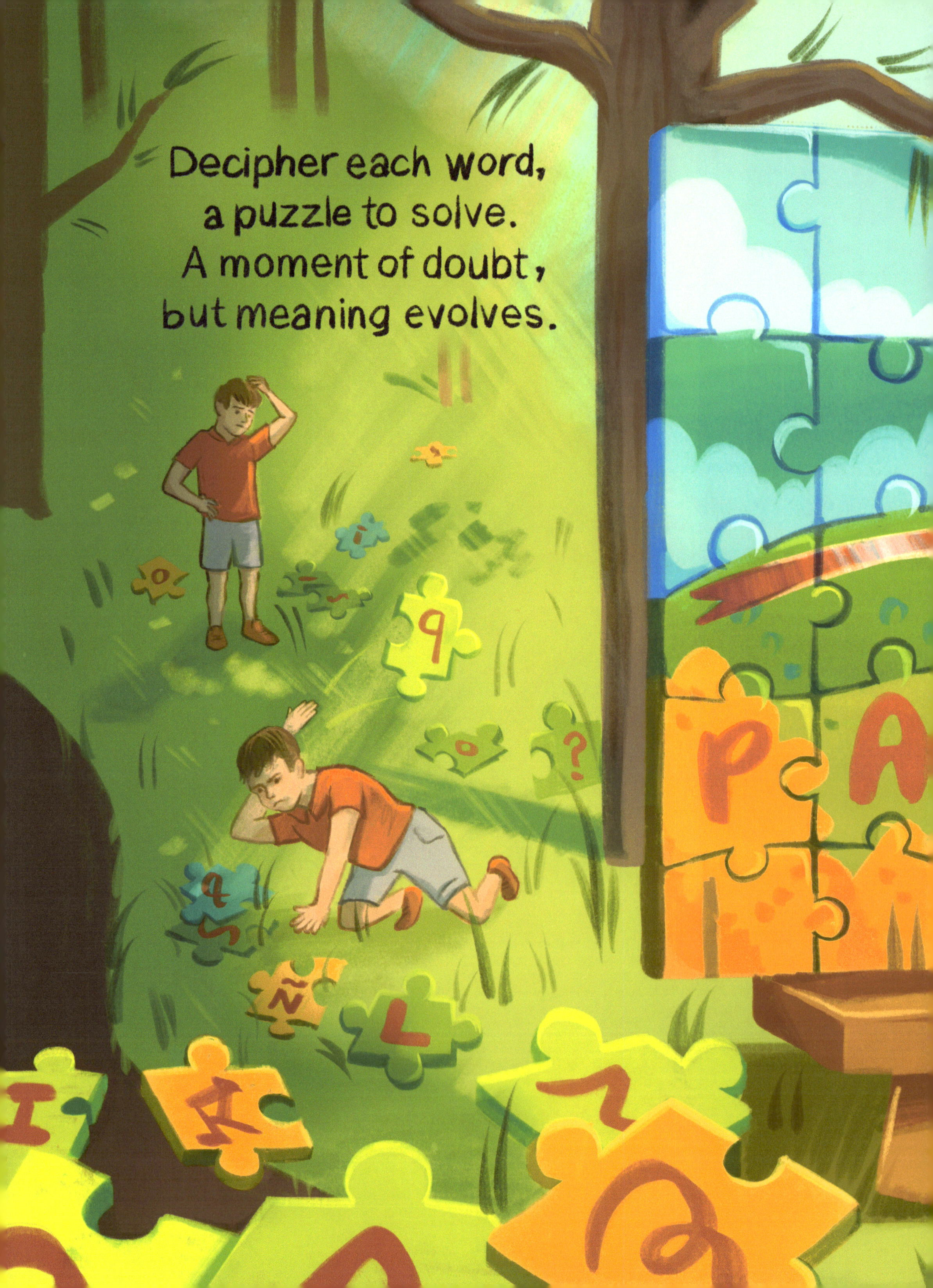

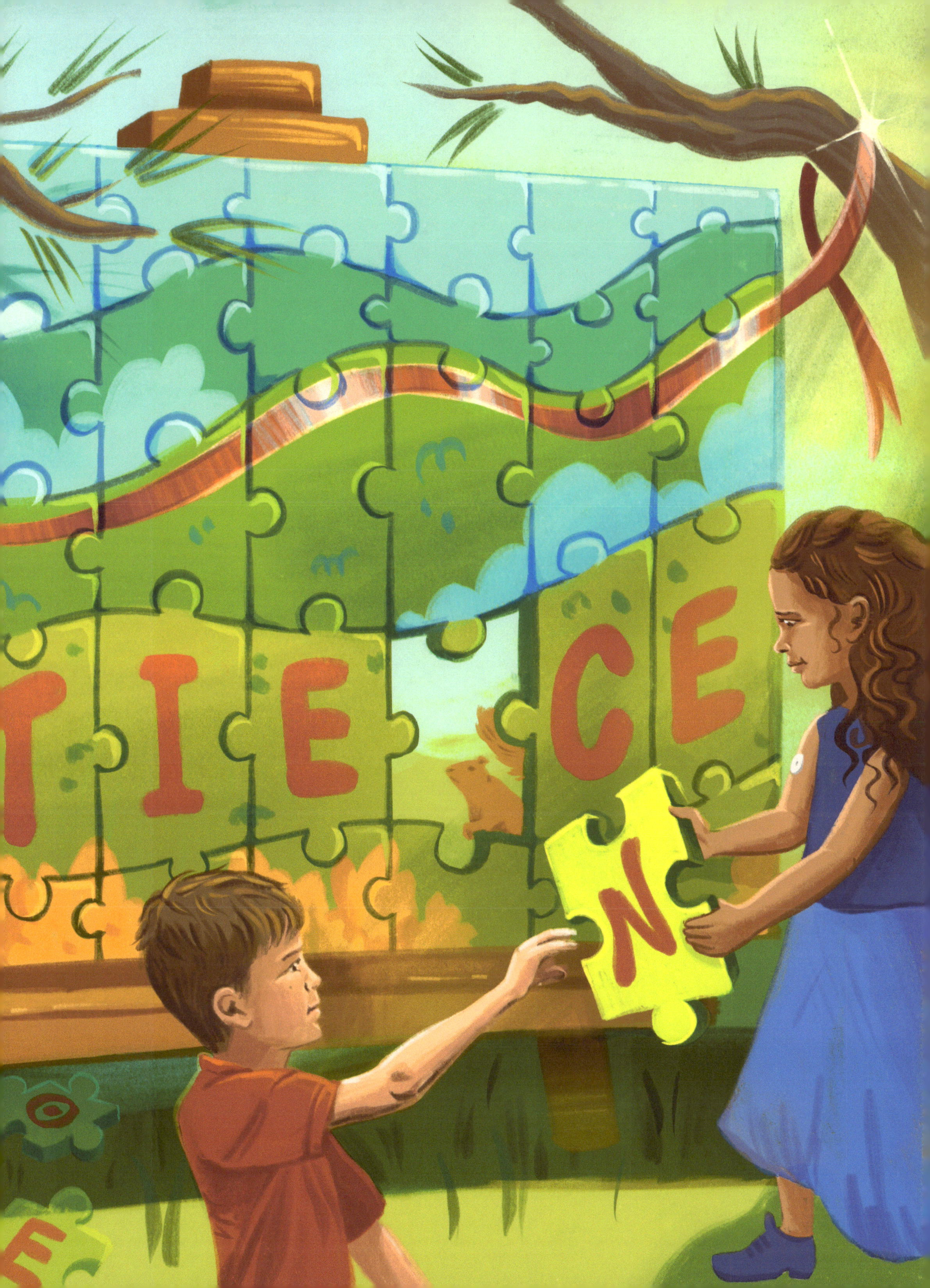
TIE
CE
N

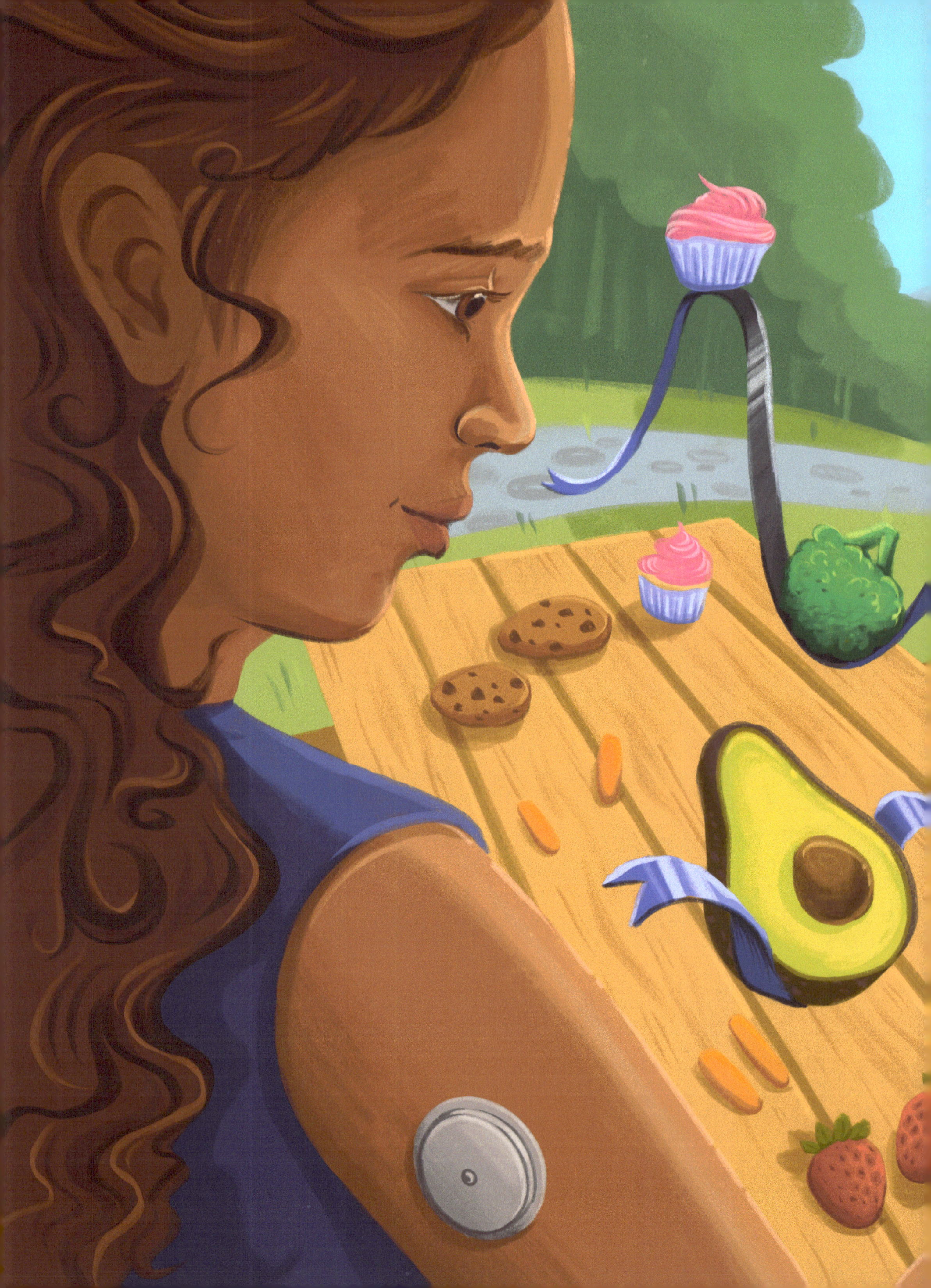

Soaring high or low,
levels will vary.
Like the changing winds,
the strand will carry.

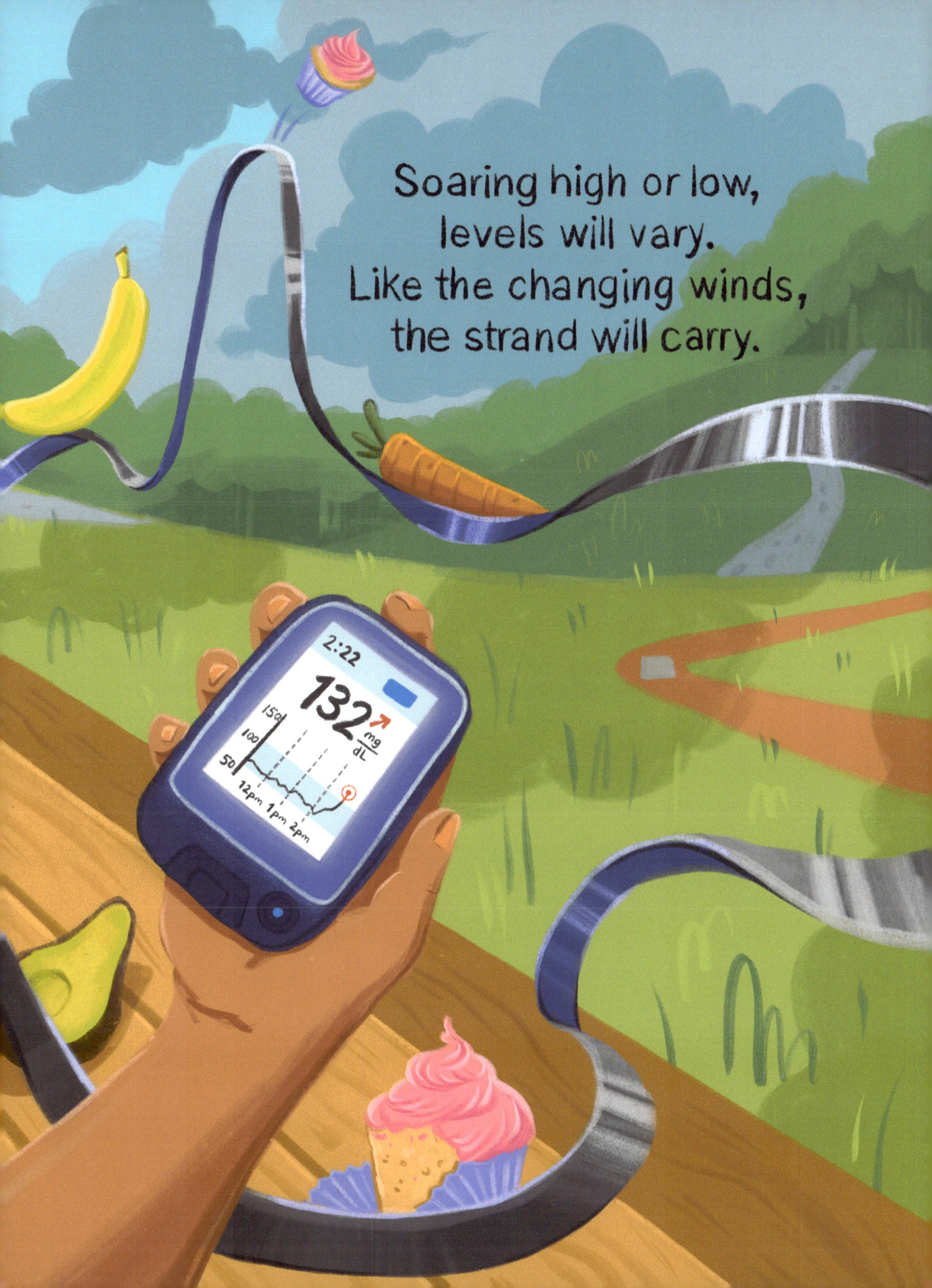

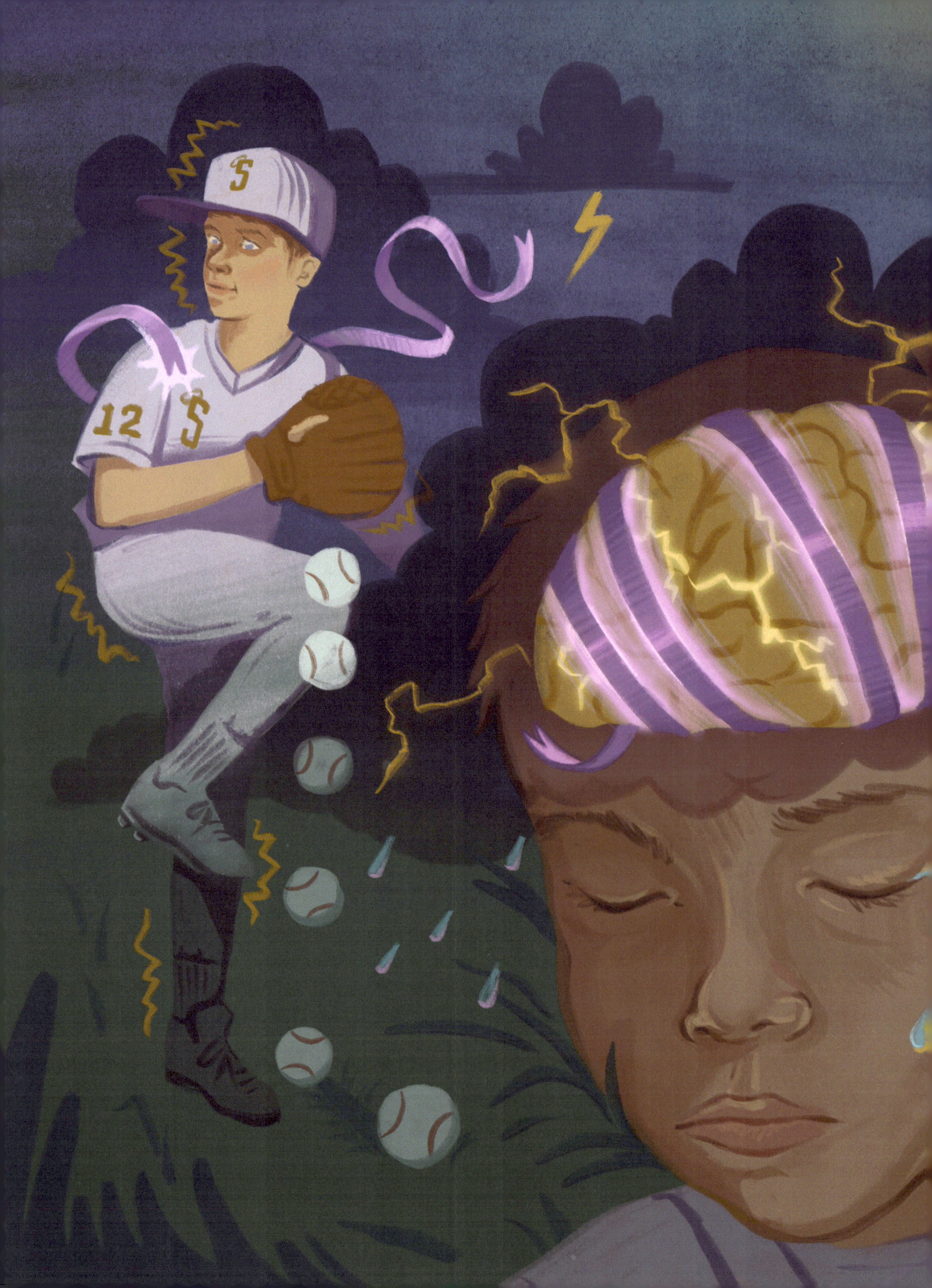

The unknown of when–
And nothing to control.
Resting by your side,
let the storm unfold.

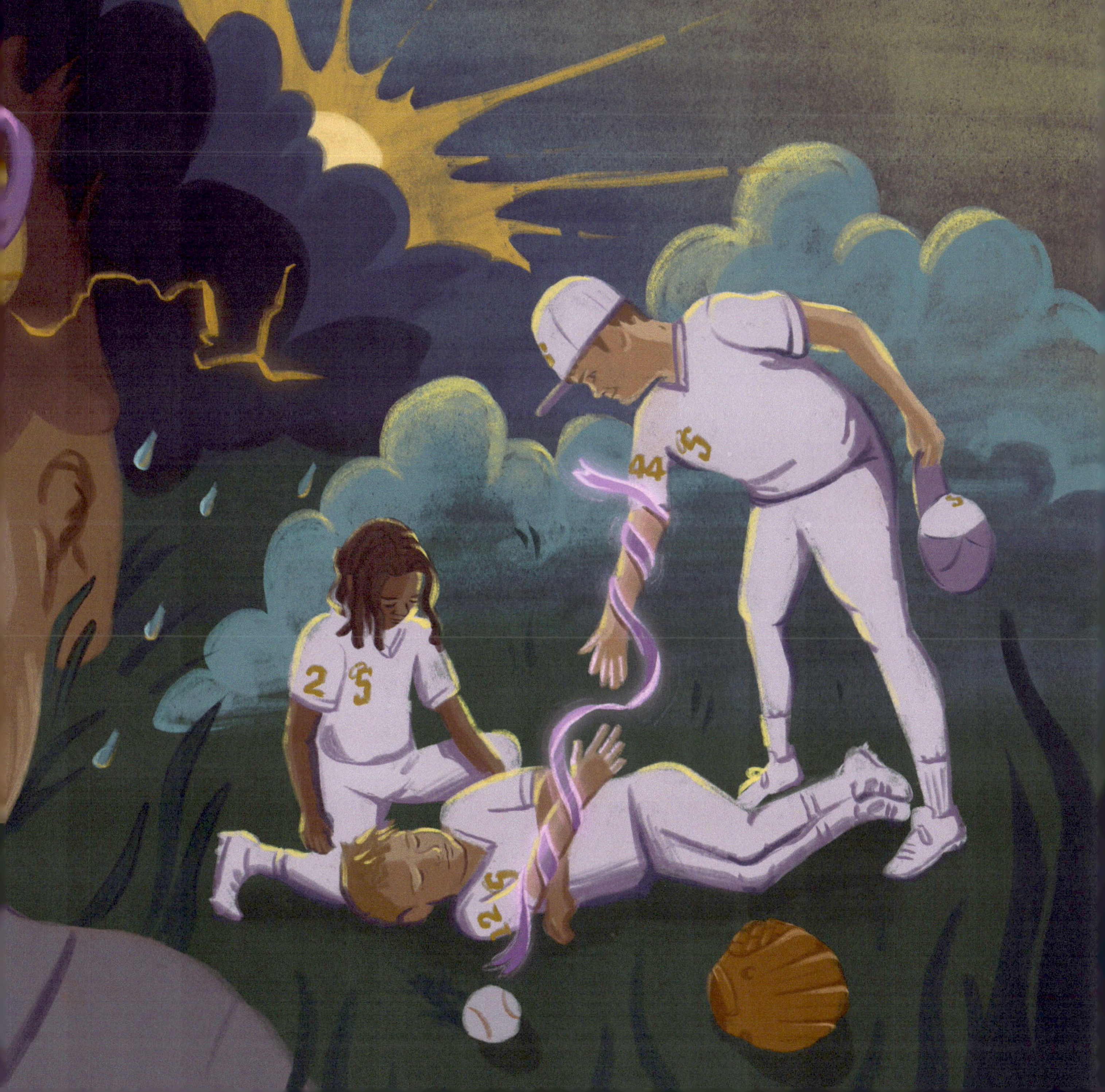

Worthy of each space;
never to confine.
Bound only by grace,
look ahead—not behind.

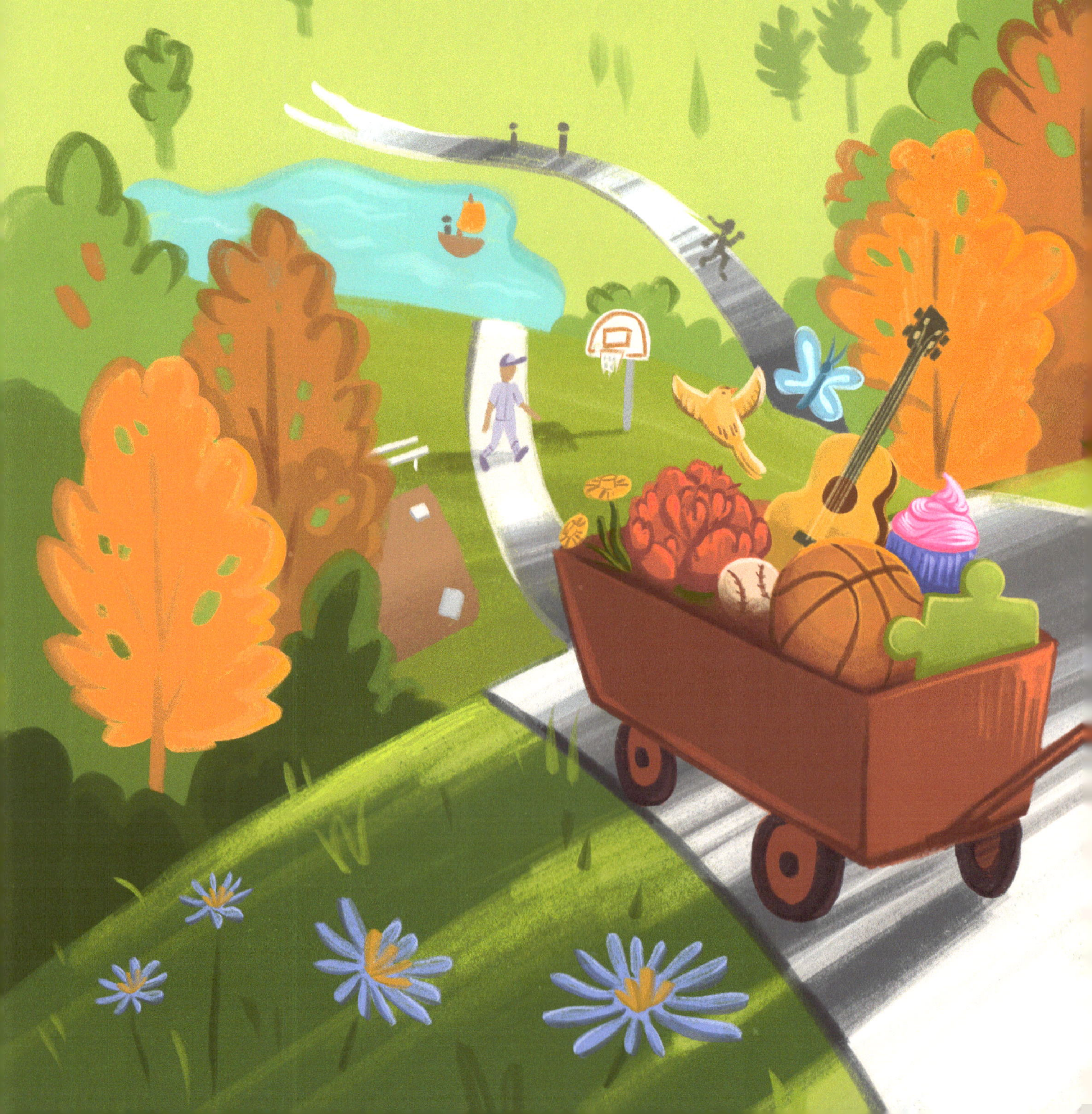

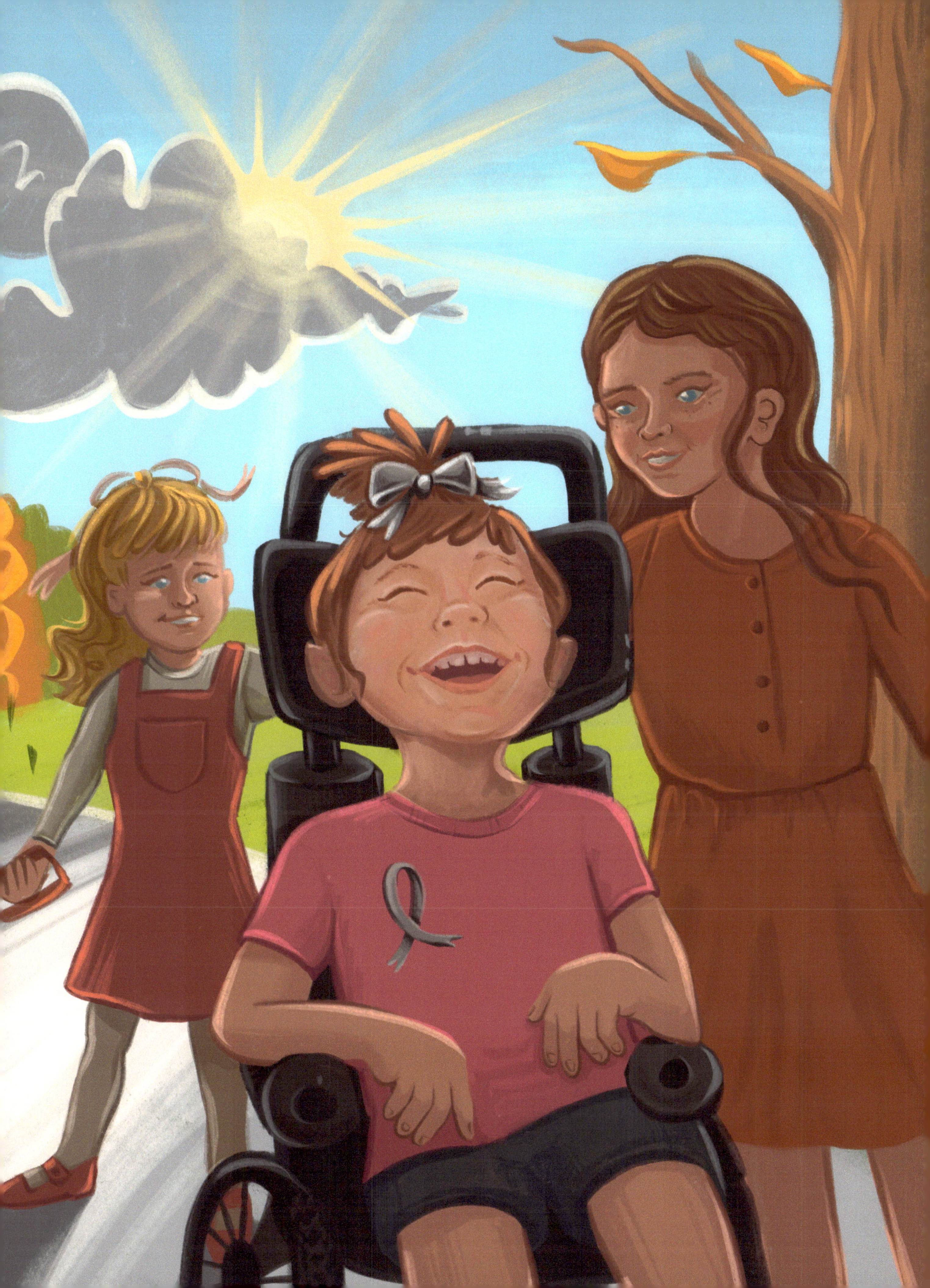

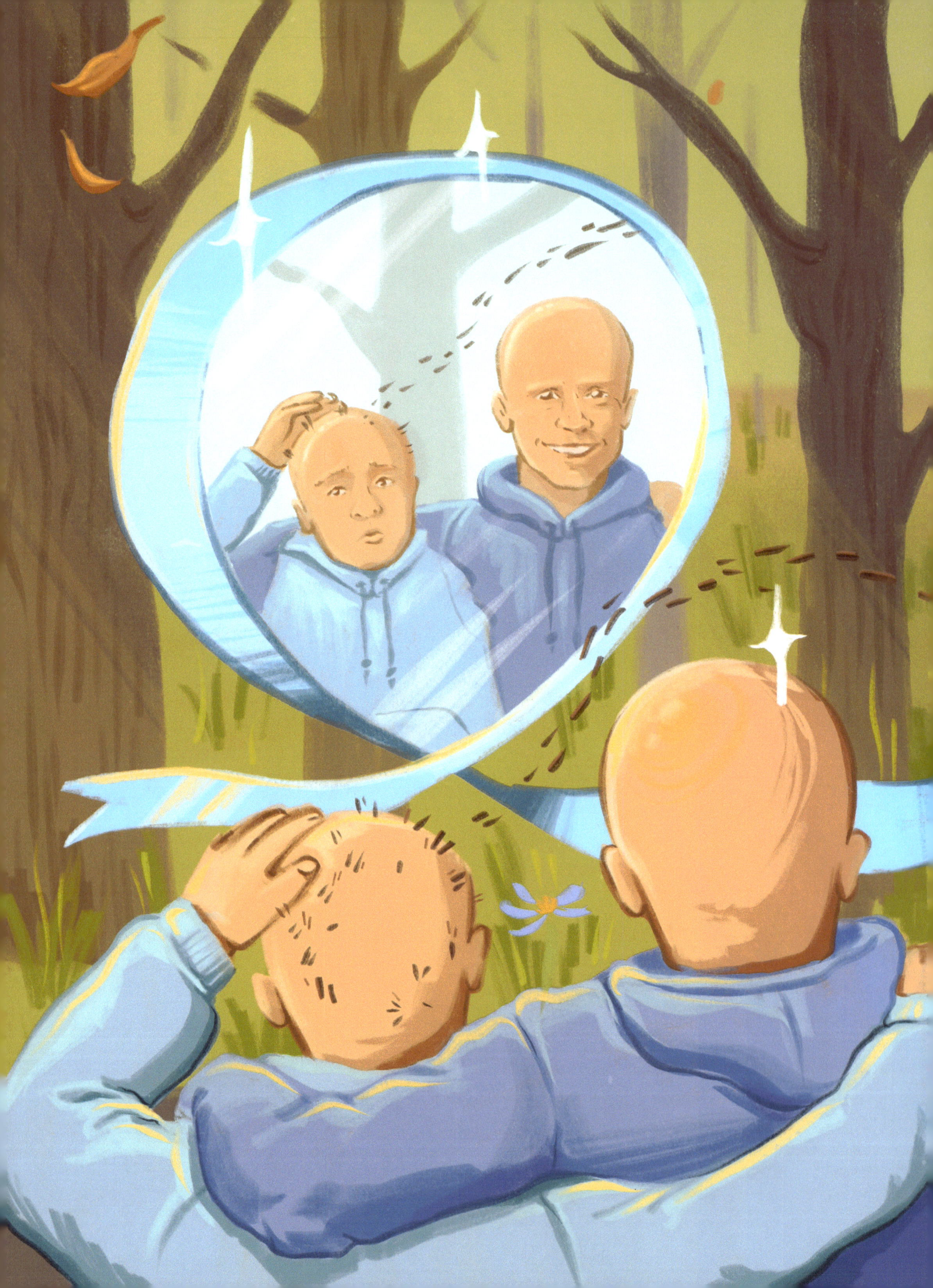

Like fallen petals,
locks of hair fall.
No shame for what's gone,
just beauty for all.

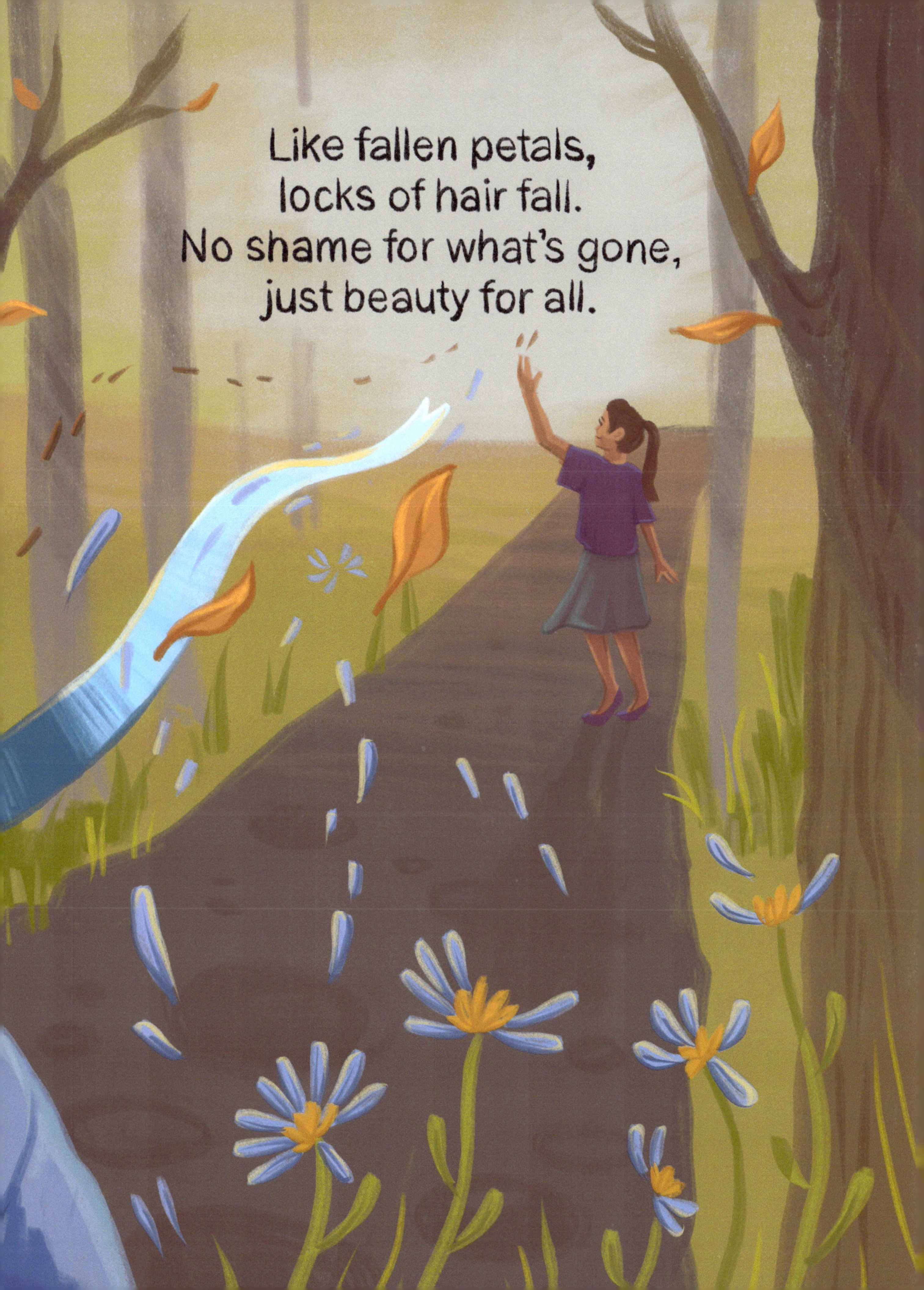

Woven in worry,
time given to care.
A loving embrace
for what you must bear.

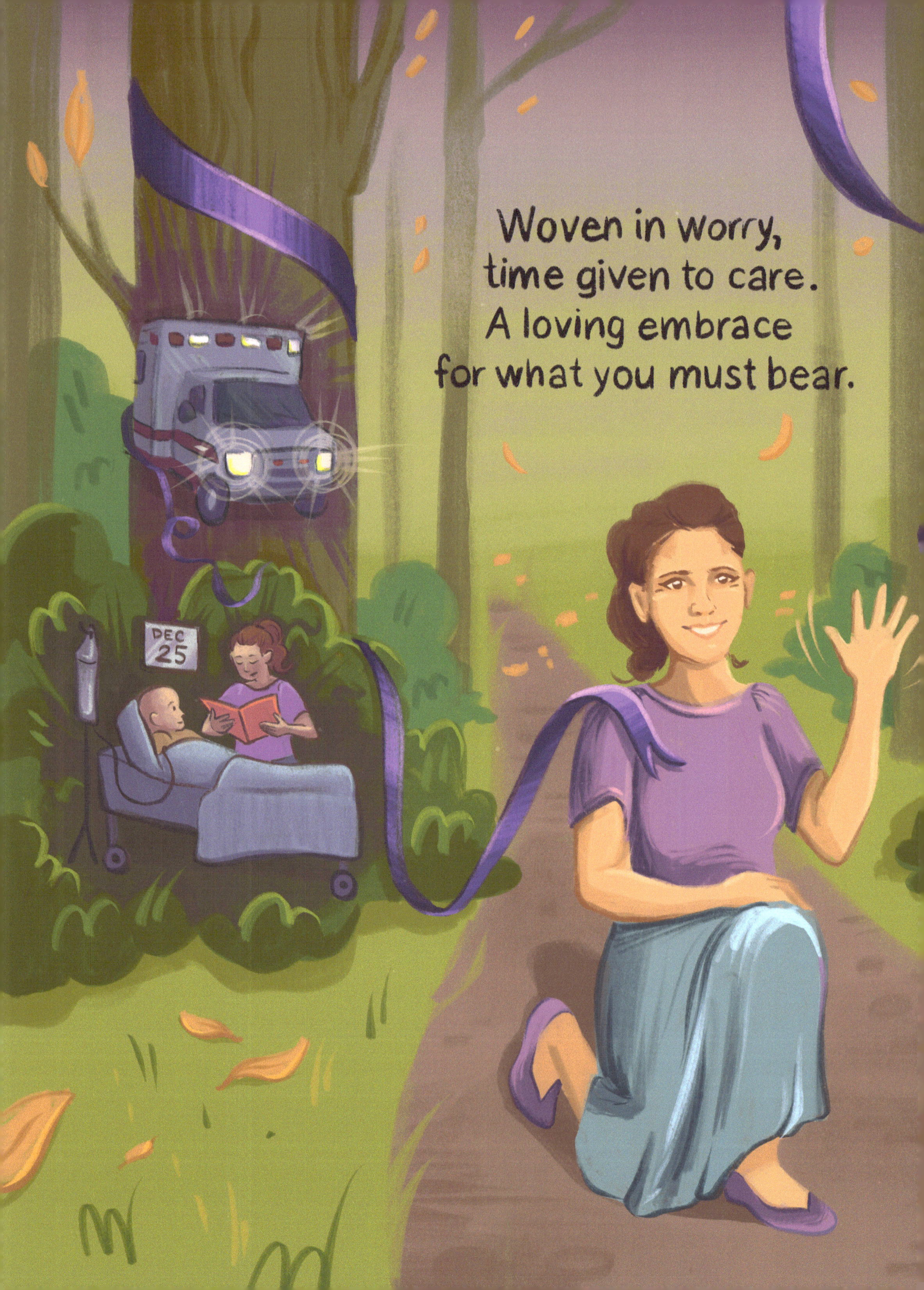

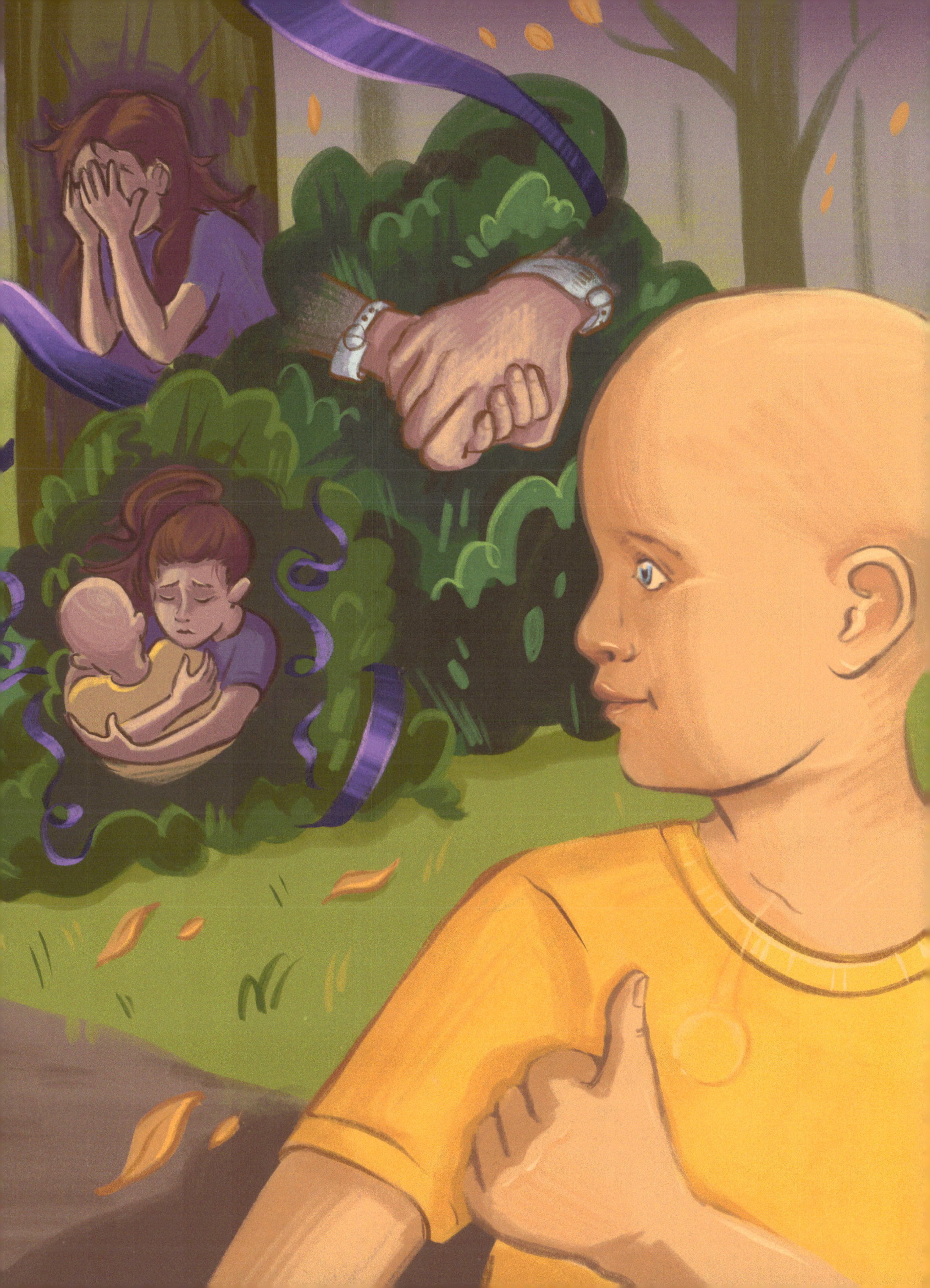

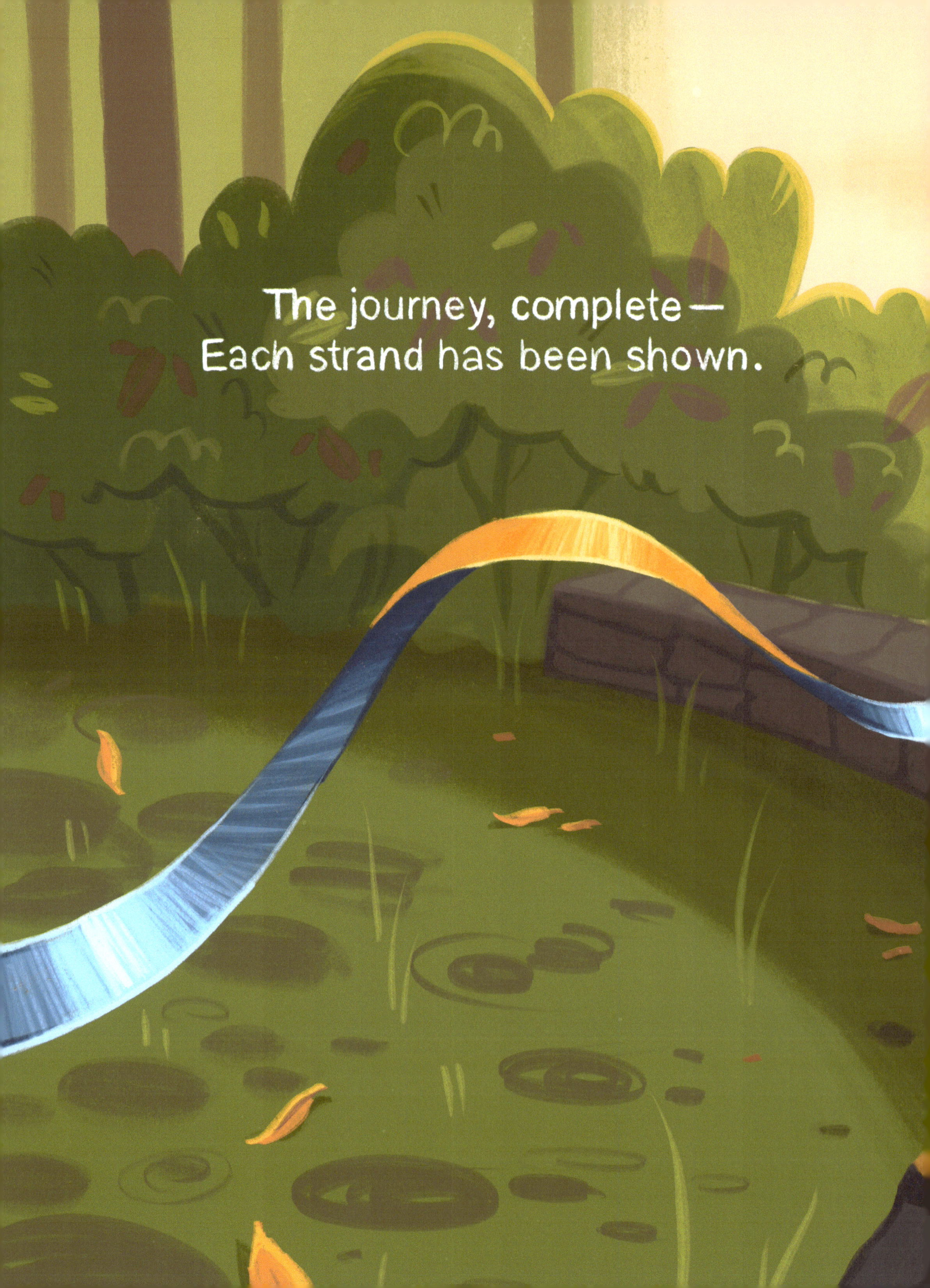

The journey, complete—
Each strand has been shown.

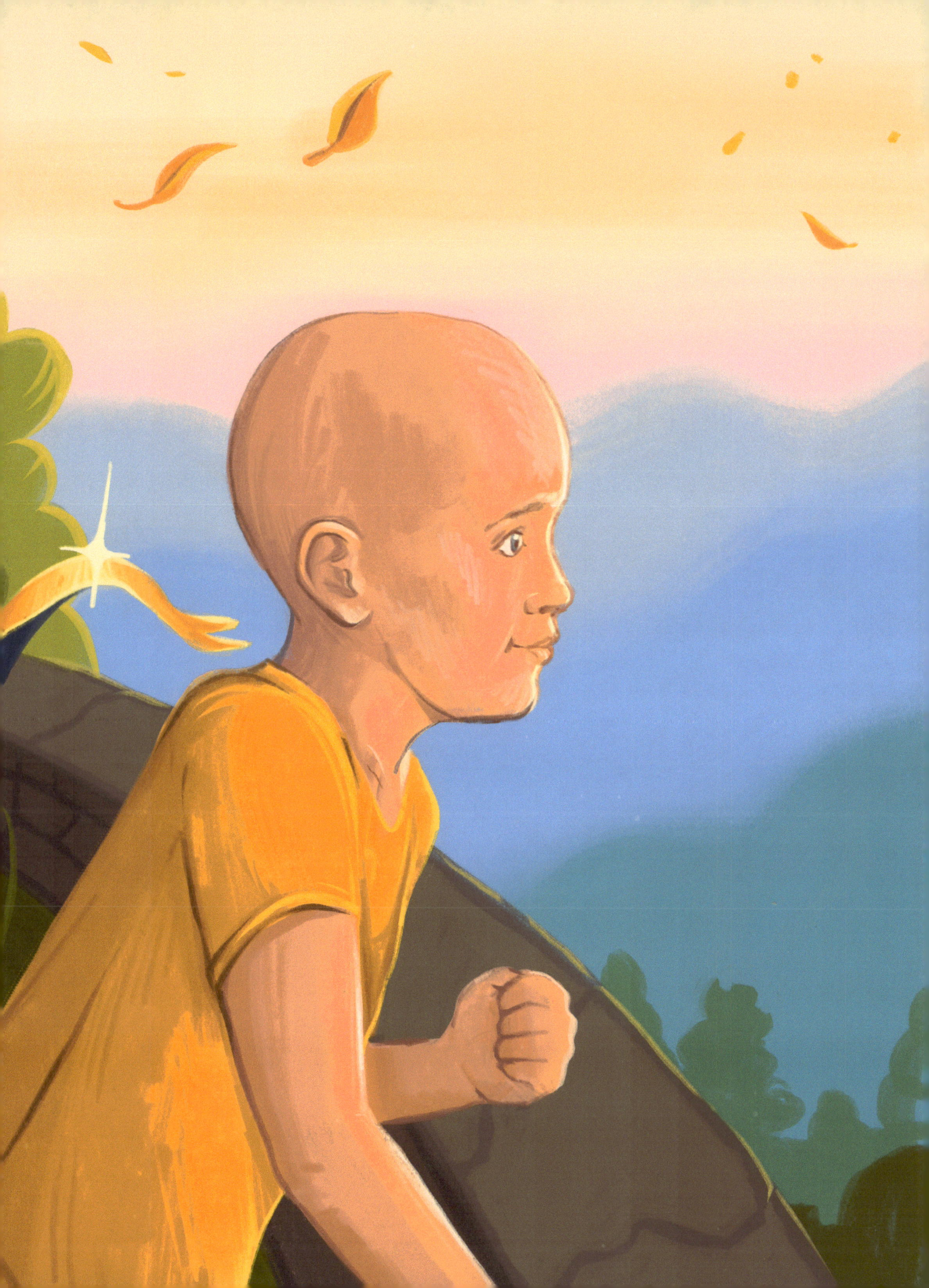

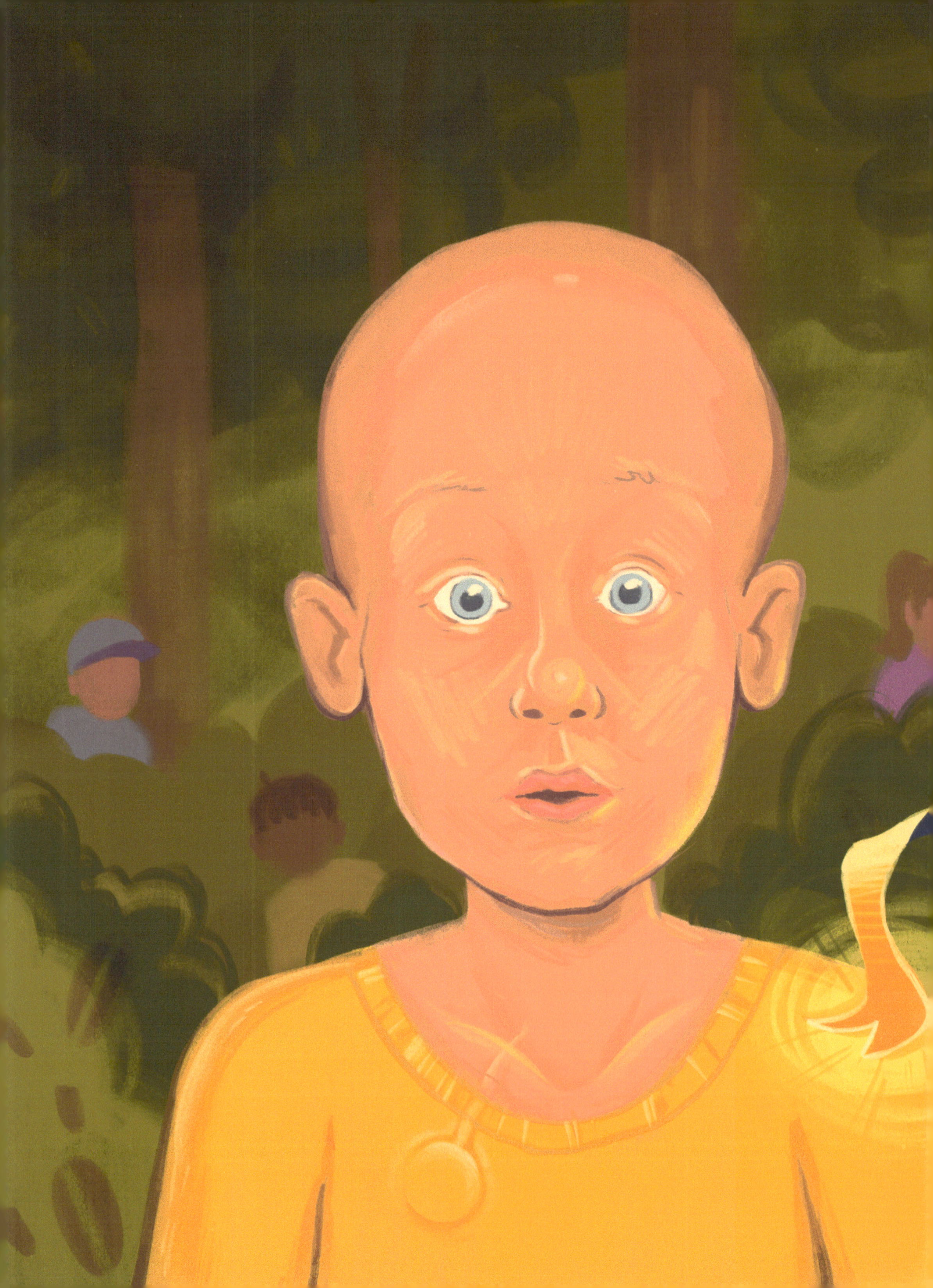

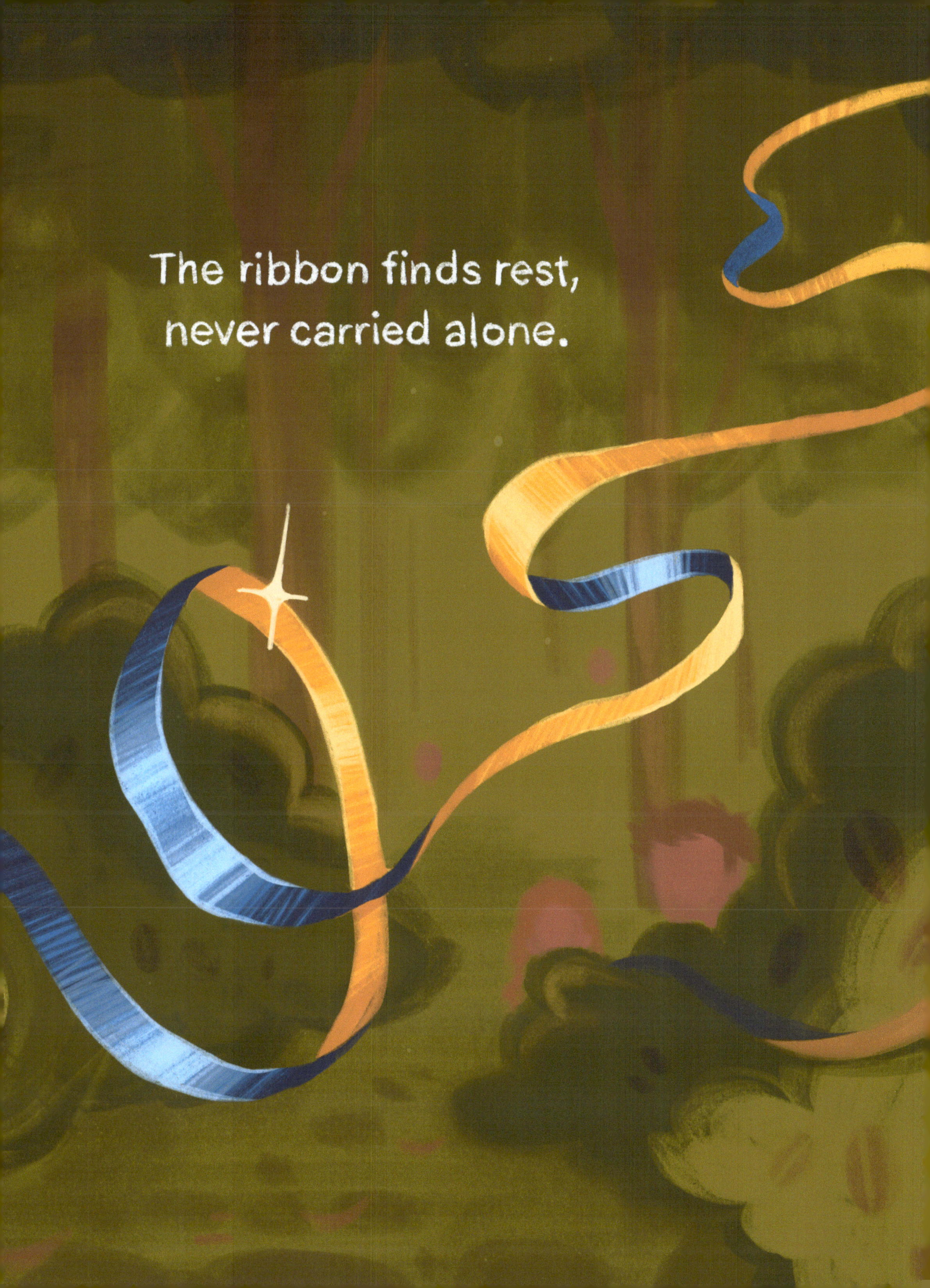

The ribbon finds rest,
never carried alone.

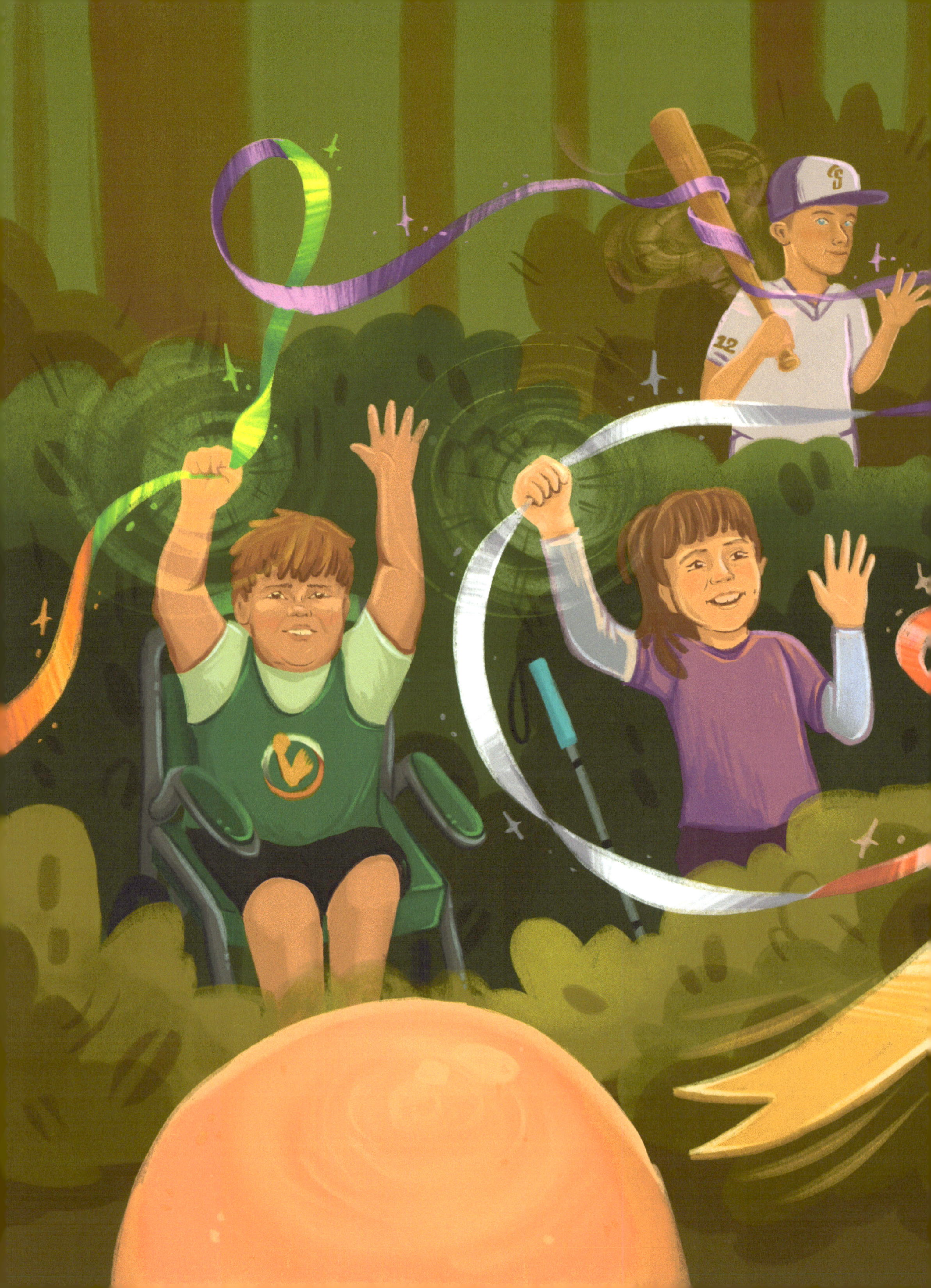
12

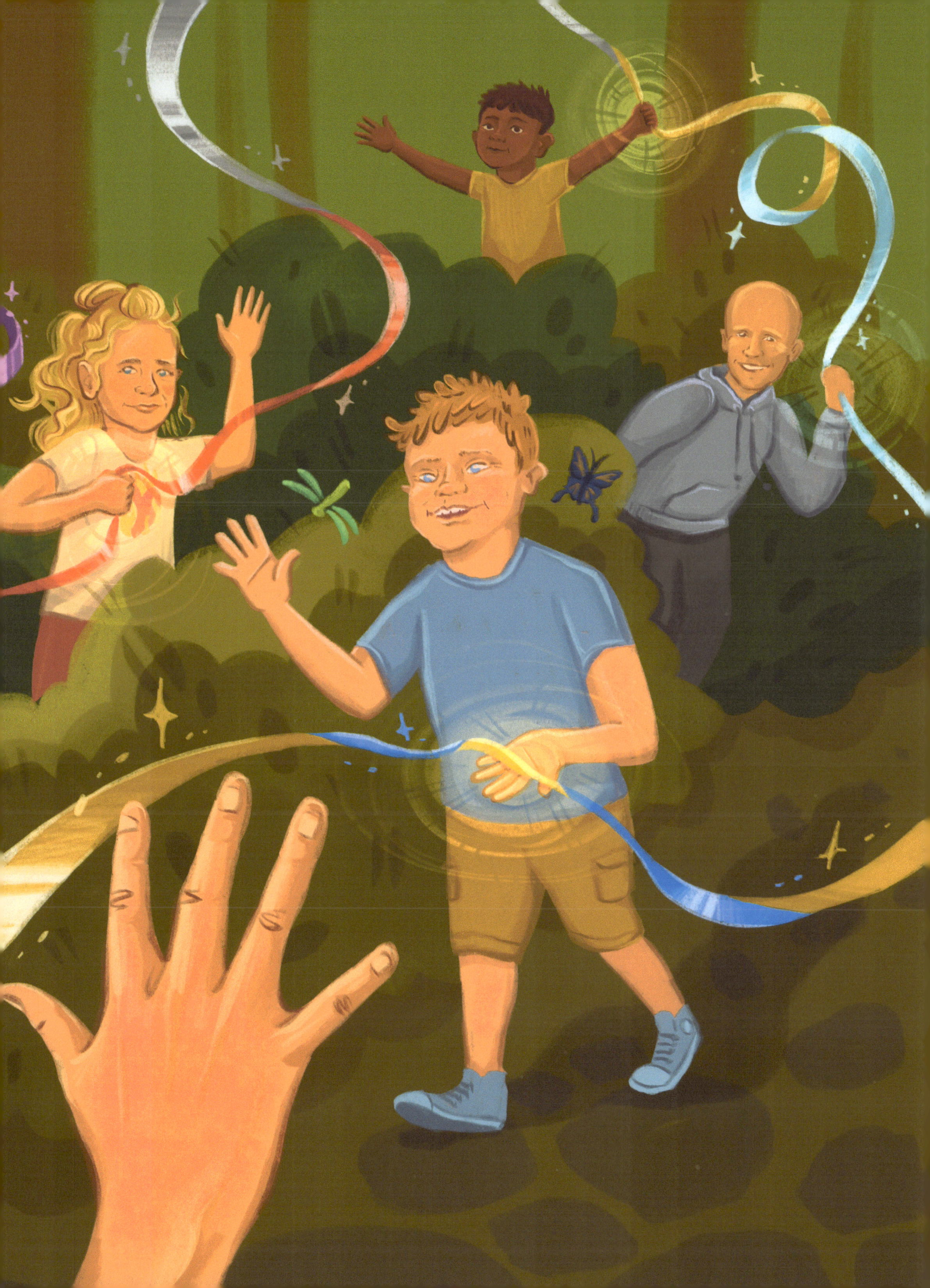

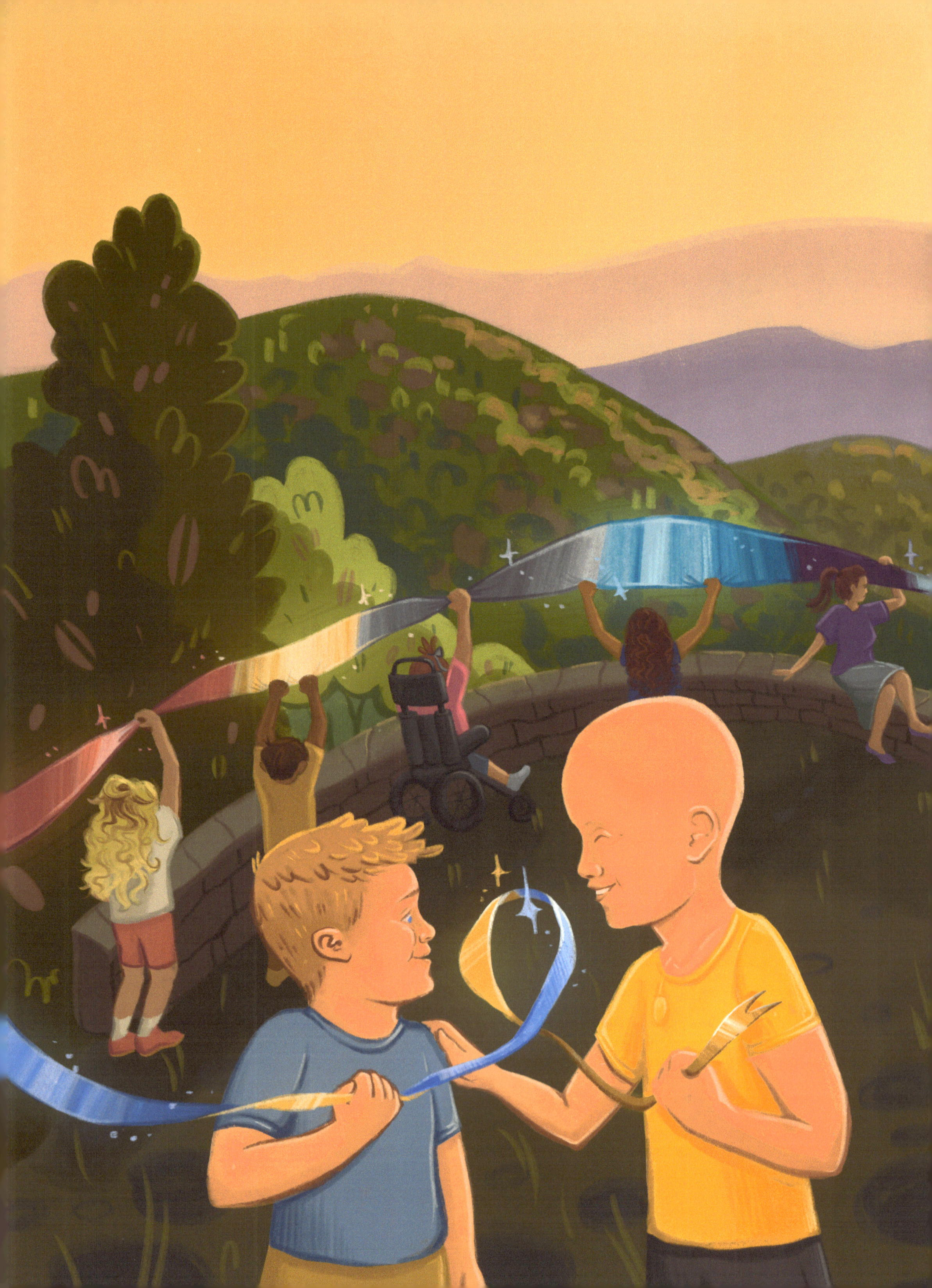

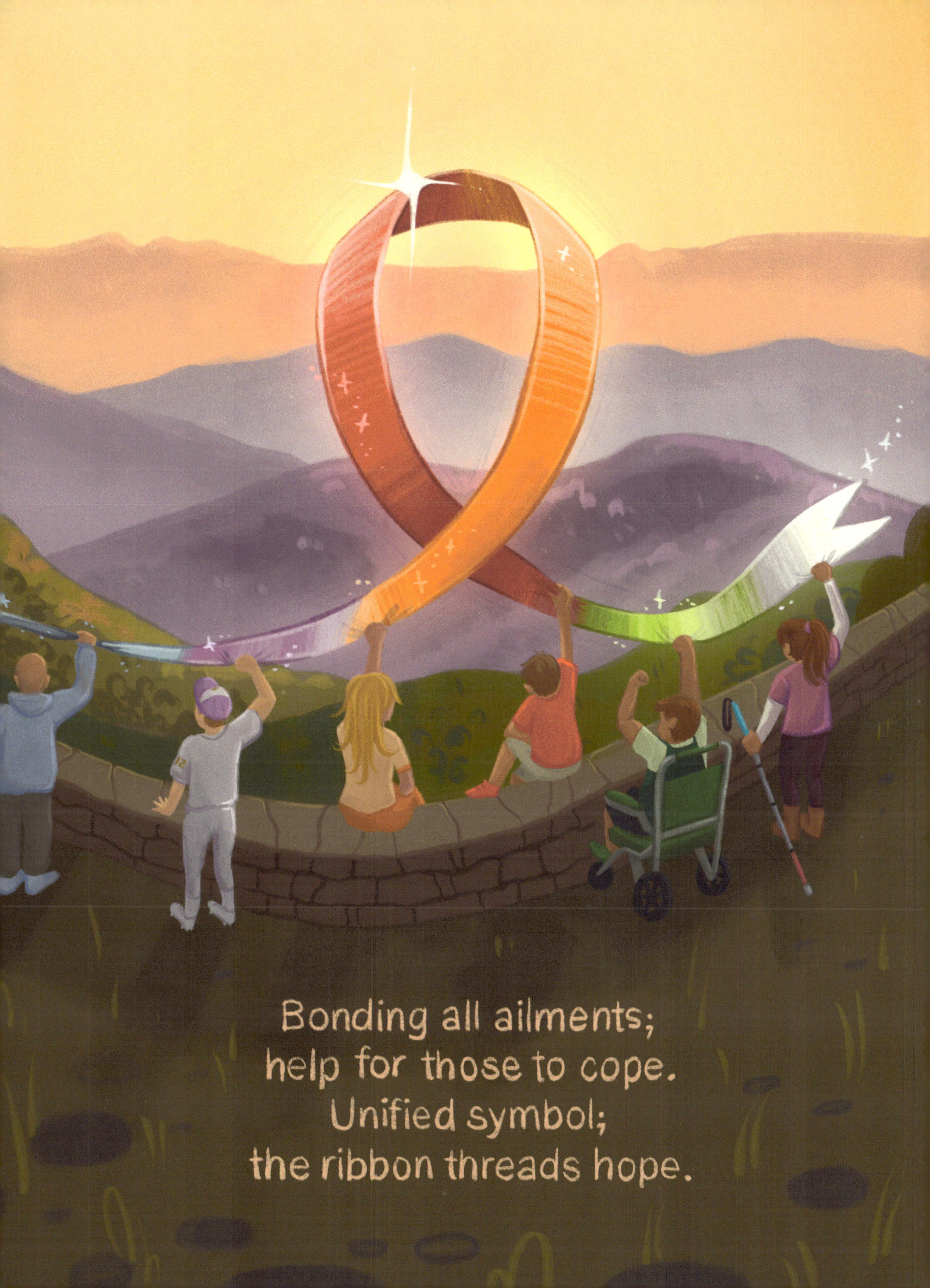

Bonding all ailments;
help for those to cope.
Unified symbol;
the ribbon threads hope.

You are
loved.

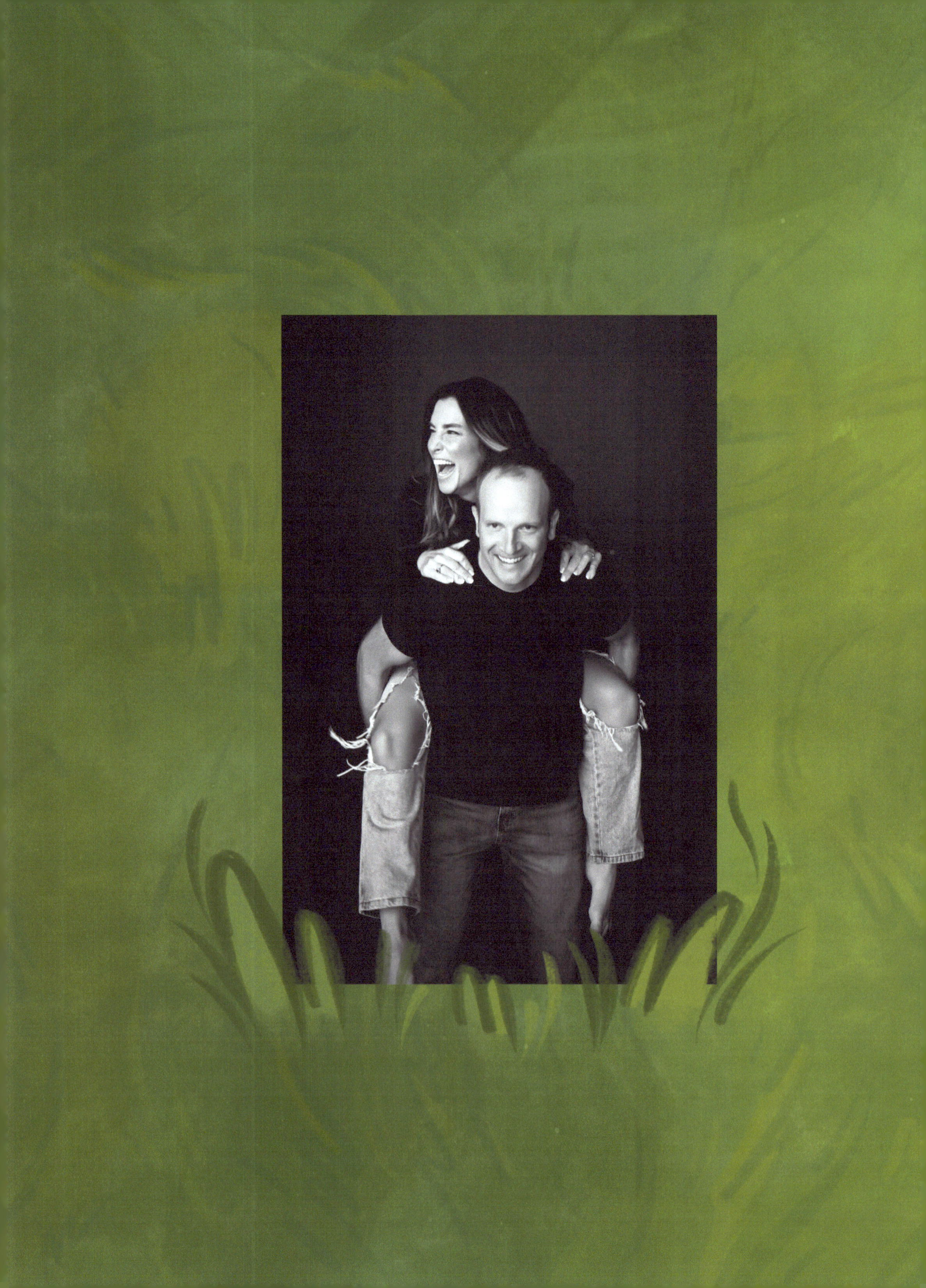

The following back matter section was co-authored by Dr. Jamie Seidl and Beth Seidl. Dr. Jamie Seidl served as a United States Army Family Practice Physician and currently serves as a medical director at the VA Hospital in Des Moines, Iowa. We extend our deepest appreciation to those children and parents who bravely shared their stories, helping deepen our understanding of the realities of their diagnosis.

CANCER

Gold

Leukemias are the most common childhood cancers. Childhood or pediatric cancer describes a group of cancers in children from infancy to 18 years old. Leukemias are cancers of bone marrow and blood. Other pediatric cancers include cancer of the brain, spinal cord, kidneys, muscle, bone, eye, and immune system lymphomas.

Children who have been diagnosed can endure treatments such as chemotherapy, radiation, immunotherapy, bone marrow transplant, or surgery. Some patients will have a port surgically placed. This is a small device that is positioned just under the skin and used for administering treatments like chemotherapy. Common side effects of these treatments can include hair loss, fatigue, flu-like symptoms, or make someone more prone to be hospitalized or ill from the common cold.

According to the National Cancer Institute, pediatric cancer mortality rates have seen a substantial drop in the past fifty years. Current mortality rates are 2.2 per 100,000 pediatric cancer patients. This rate stems from advancements in detection and diagnoses along with targeted cancer treatments. Continued early detection occurs with the help of parents, family members, and doctors who may recognize symptoms such as easy bruising or bleeding, swelling, unexplained weight loss, or fevers.

A Specialist often involved in your care:
Hematologist or Oncologist

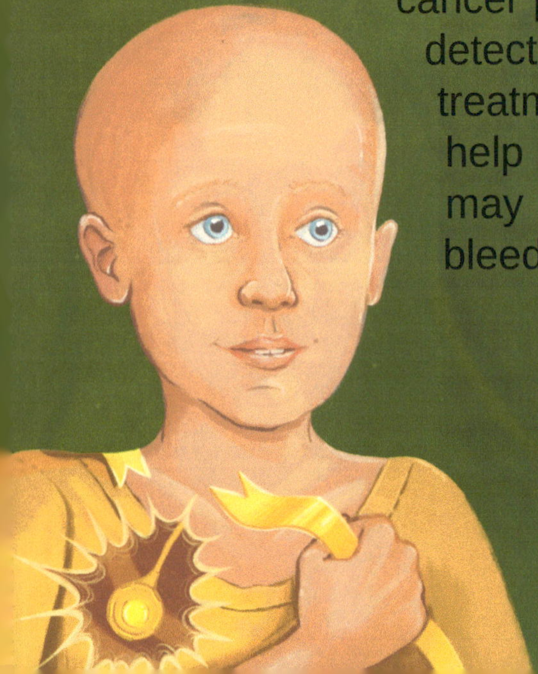

Patient Perspective:

Johnathan and William
(answered by their mother, Kaitlin)

What is something other kids should understand about Cancer?

Kaitlin (Johnathan and William): Cancer is NOT contagious… Most of society feels familiar with cancer, but navigating the world with a body facing challenges is entirely different. Cancer seems scary because the treatments can make the body hurt, make people feel sick, and cause them to lose hair. Adults tend to treat children as fragile and in need of extra protection, even after treatment. This can be very alienating, especially when a child's identity is tied to an illness or disability by others.

What helps you feel seen or supported?

Kaitlin (Johnathan and William): I shared pictures and writing long ago to keep people updated, and to offer encouragement and education along the way. It built connections and showed me how many people were offering tangible support. Every card, text, or message that someone is thinking of us matters.

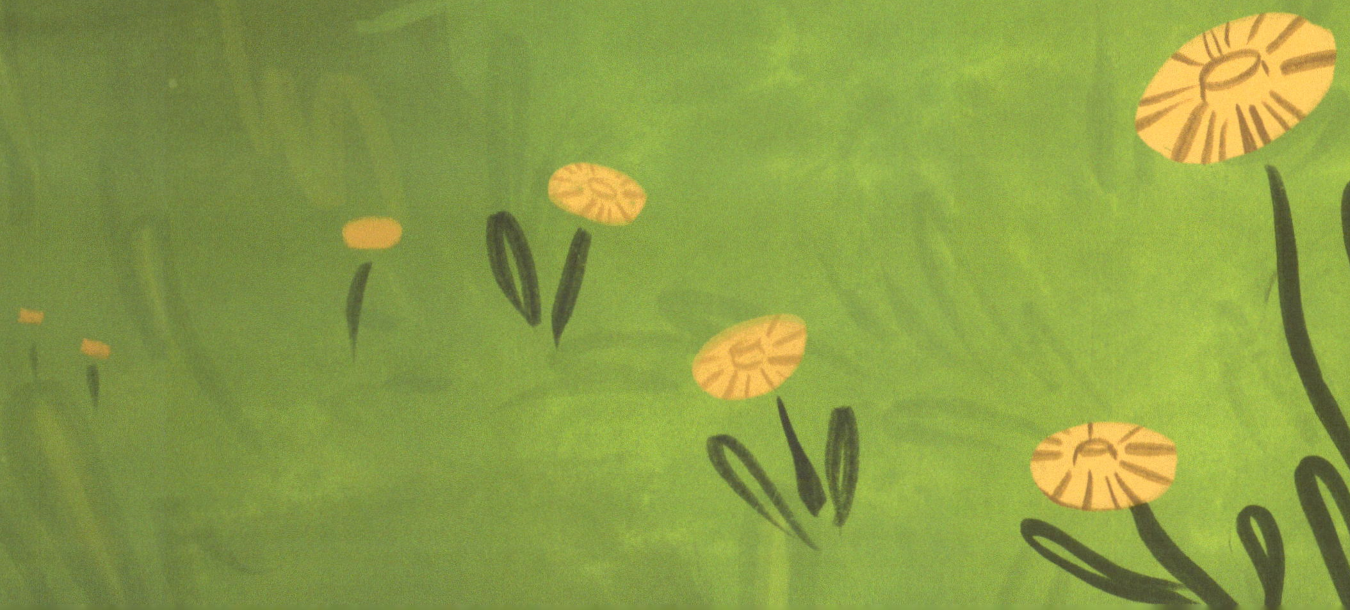

DOWN SYNDROME

Blue & Yellow

Down Syndrome encompasses a genetic disorder where a child receives an extra copy of chromosome 21. Chromosomes are a DNA blueprint that helps design everything about us: from the way our ears, eyes, and nose are shaped to the way in which we can learn and communicate. Unique physical features can include but are not limited to an upslanting of the eyelids, an excess skin fold on the inner corners of the eyes, flattened nasal bridge, low set or small folded ears, short neck, protruding tongue, incurved fifth finger, or transverse palmar crease.

Other conditions or complications related to Down Syndrome may include congenital heart disease, gastrointestinal tract abnormalities, cognitive impairments, lower growth trajectories, visual and hearing impairments, thyroid disorder, diabetes, hematological abnormalities, respiratory conditions, skin disorders, infertility, hypermobility of joints, or immunologic impairments.

With the help of a developmental pediatrician, patients are able to build a network of team members to support both the patient and family members. Despite their numerous ailments, children with Down Syndrome often possess a positive worldview with outward displays of emotions that captivate those around them.

A Specialist often involved in your care:
Developmental-Behavioral Pediatrician

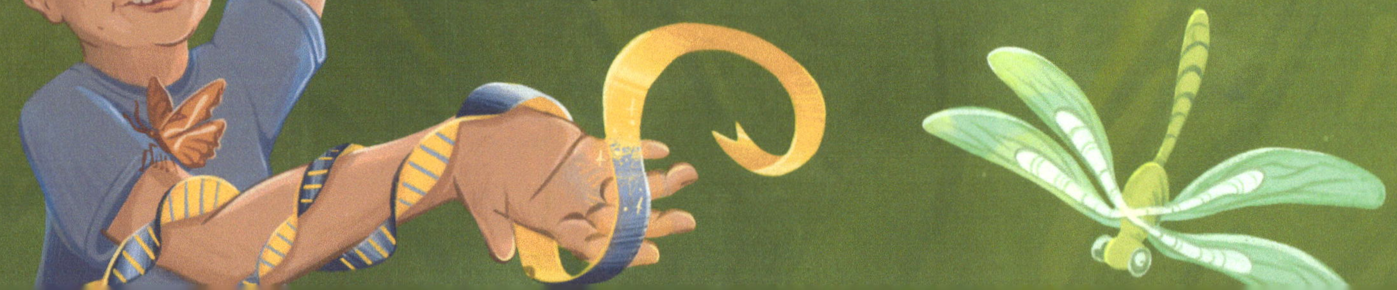

Patient Perspective:

William (answered by his mother, Kaitlin)
and Lincoln

What is something other kids should understand about Down Syndrome?

Kaitlin (William): Kids with Down Syndrome understand they are different and want to be included. There is so much more to the individual than what help may be needed. Down Syndrome is also a spectrum; some may function very independently, while others need much more substantial help. It is important not to infantilize people or assume they lack intelligence because they look or speak differently.

Lincoln: We live each day to the fullest—smile, smile, smile!

What helps you feel seen or supported?

Kaitlin (William): Media representation is so meaningful! Seeing actors and actresses with Down Syndrome in the media, modeling in advertisements, included in school photo proofs, etc. creates an equality most don't consider. When friends, family, and community members willingly learn more about Down Syndrome, raise awareness, participate in events, and educate others, it feels like our loved ones will be safer in the world.

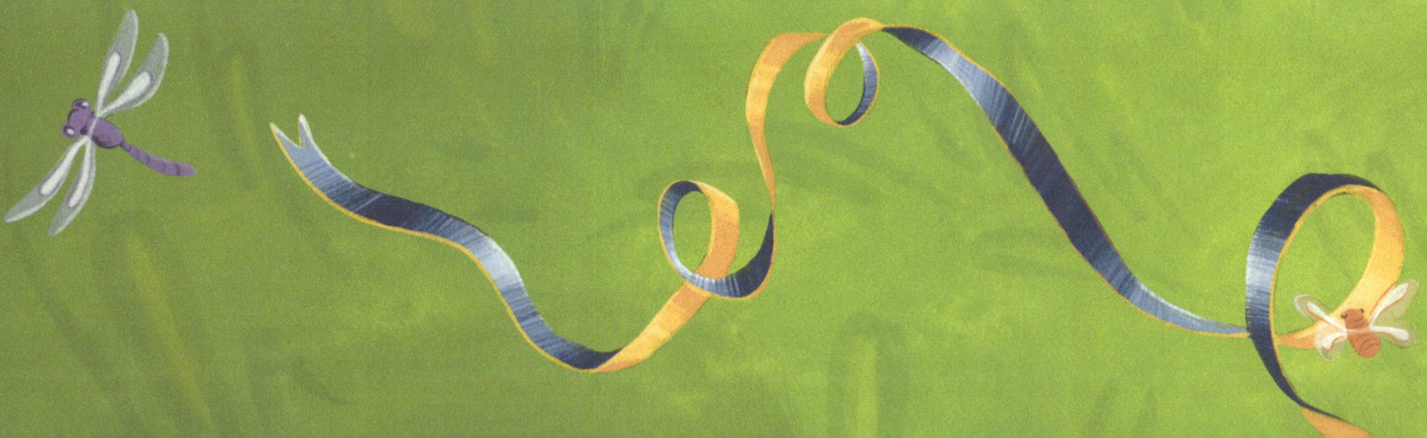

HEART DISORDERS

Red

A grouping of disorders that affect the heart and its ability to function properly. These conditions can present with symptoms of fatigue due to the inability to properly pump oxygenated blood to the body.

This can present as early as infancy if babies have a difficult time nursing or feeding. Children with these conditions have a hard time receiving enough oxygen, resulting in cyanosis or blue discoloration.

Children or adolescents may be diagnosed due to activity intolerance, poor weight gain, syncope, or heart murmurs found on a heart exam. Diagnosis is found through a detailed physical examination, electrocardiography (ECG), chest x-ray, vital signs (blood pressure, heart rate, and pulse oxygenation), and advanced imaging such as an echocardiogram. An ECG is commonly obtained in children with heart conditions and entails connecting leads to capture the electrical activity of the heart.

Treatment depends on the stability of the patient. Imaging and procedures are often repeated as the child grows and develops. Many children may have to take heart medications for the rest of their lives. Heart disorders can also prevent children from fully participating in activities due to the risk of sudden cardiac failure.

A Specialist often involved in your care: **Cardiologist**

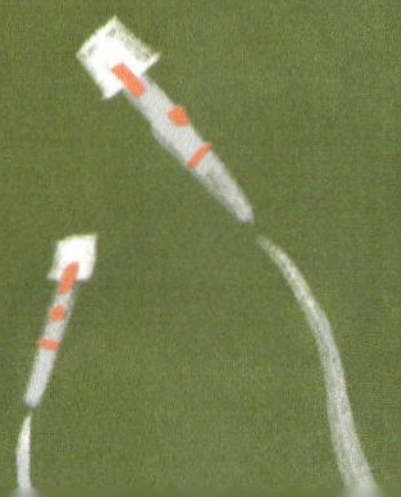

Patient Perspective:

Emily
(answered by her mother, Heather)

What is something other kids should understand about your heart condition?

Heather (Emily): A heart condition is invisible. You can't see it. Our hearts are meant to beat faster when we are doing a workout or exerting a lot of energy, but my heart beats even faster than a normal heart that works hard. A heart isn't built to sustain beating that fast so the muscle wears out, causing my heart issue.

What helps you feel seen or supported?

Heather (Emily): We understand it is hard to leave a child with a medical condition because people are scared to babysit your child. The logistics of leaving Emily have gotten easier as she has grown older, but we still have our reservations any time we leave or have another event for her sisters. I often find myself thinking the other shoe hasn't dropped and I am trying to prepare myself for what's next. The best way to support us is showing up not only for Emily, but her sisters. Whether it is a long hospital stay or surgery, dropping off dinner or picking up the other siblings, those moments of help and kindness mean the most.

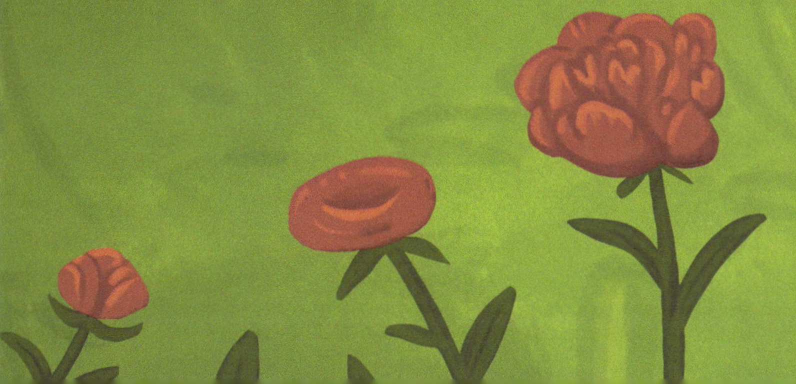

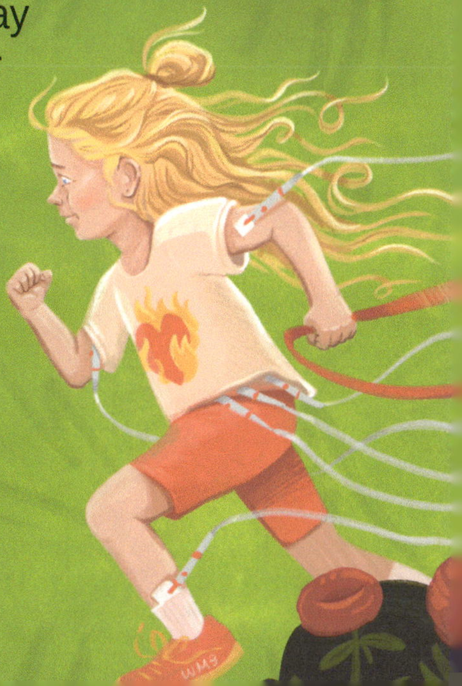

VISUAL IMPAIRMENT

White

The leading cause of childhood blindness is retinopathy of prematurity. Retinopathy of prematurity affects 31.3% of the population of blind children. Other causes of blindness include trauma, infection, nutritional deficiencies, inflammation, genetics, cancer, and a variety of eye disorders. Visual impairments may cause delays in social, emotional, and learning development.

Childhood refractive errors are a common health condition that affects up to 25% of children ages 5-17. Refractive errors are disorders of the eye structures and occur when images are not properly focused on the eyes' retina, resulting in blurred vision.

Myopia (nearsightedness), hyperopia (farsightedness), and astigmatism are the three types of refractive errors.

Children at school may experience sensitivity to light, blurred vision, headache, or eye strain. The most common treatments for refractive errors are either eyeglasses or contact lenses.

A Specialist often involved in your care:
Ophthalmologist

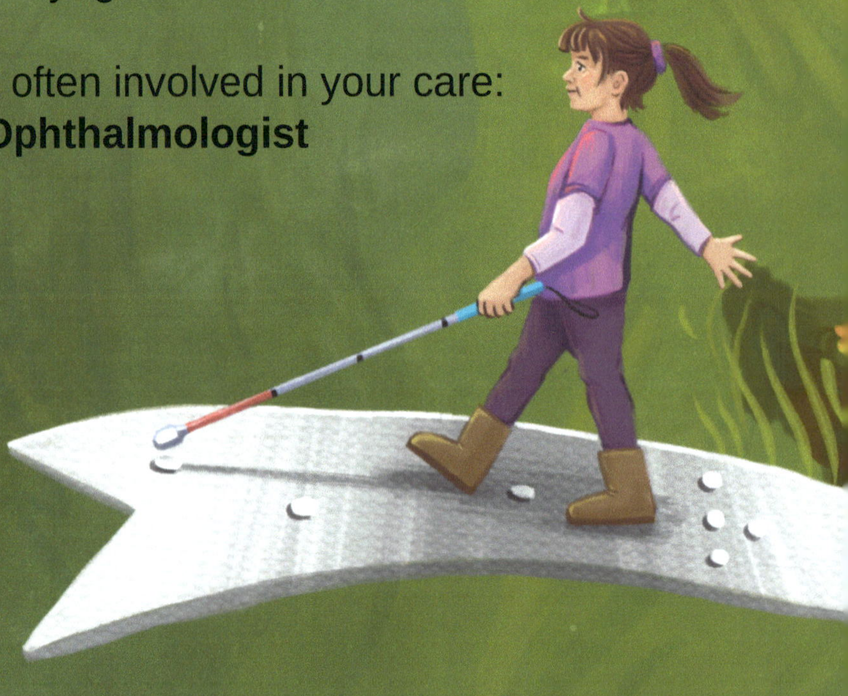

Patient Perspective:

Zoe

What is something other kids should understand about Blindness?

Zoe: Everyone assumes my entire world is dark. That may be true in the medical sense, but for me, my life is full of color. My imagination is endless and there is never a moment where I don't 'see' the beautiful colors around me. My blindness has offered me the ability to paint the world without rules or limitations. Additionally, many people think I am unable to do normal day-to-day activities. I can hold a job. I can cross the street without assistance. I can live a normal life with adaptations that keep me safe.

What helps you feel seen or supported?

Zoe: Four simple words: 'Can I help you?' These four powerful words have helped me get across a busy intersection, or they have helped me while trying to find the correct button in an elevator. I also feel supported when businesses, recreational facilities, or public places include braille and accessible technologies that help me stay independent.

HEARING IMPAIRMENT

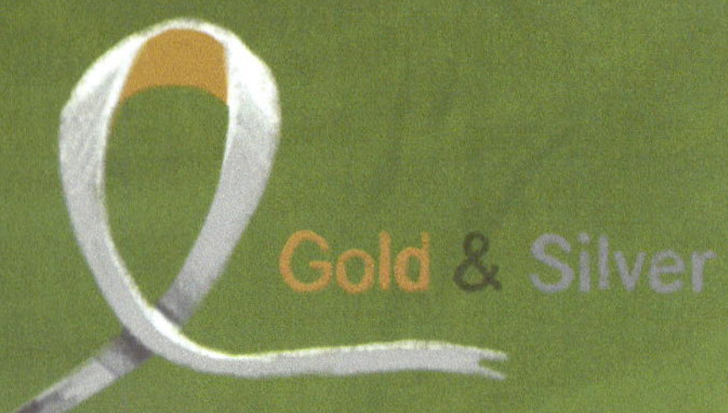

Decreased hearing or hearing loss is categorized as either conductive hearing loss or sensorineural hearing loss. Conductive hearing loss is a disorder of the middle or outer ear that impedes sound transmission to reach the inner ear. Sensorineural hearing loss stems from impairment of the inner ear to further transmit sounds appropriately to the brain.

Early recognition of hearing impairment is imperative to help reduce developmental delays. The first hearing screen occurs as a newborn before leaving the hospital—further screens may occur at school or a doctor's office. Children who are hard of hearing or deaf can experience difficulty with speech or language, learning, or social engagement.

Many resources may help support those children with hearing impairments. Interventions can provide necessary resources for the child and family members through speech therapy, occupational therapy, sign language, hearing aids, or cochlear implants.

A Specialist often involved in your care: **Otolaryngologist (ENT)**

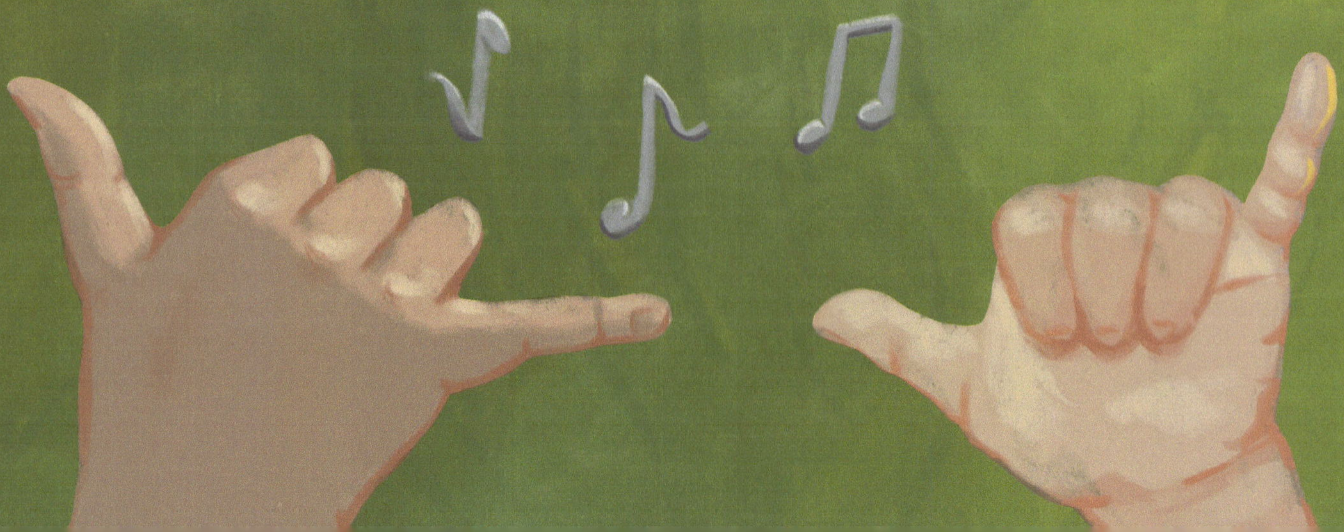

Patient Perspective:

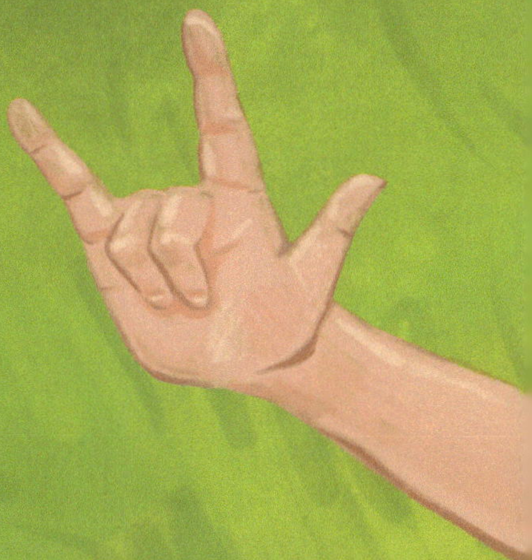

Cooper

What is something other kids should understand about Hearing Impairment or Deafness?

Cooper: I hope other kids and adults learn more sign language—I would like to talk to you. I want to be social just like every other kid.

What helps you feel seen or supported?

Cooper: I feel the most support when someone tries to learn sign language—it makes me feel included.

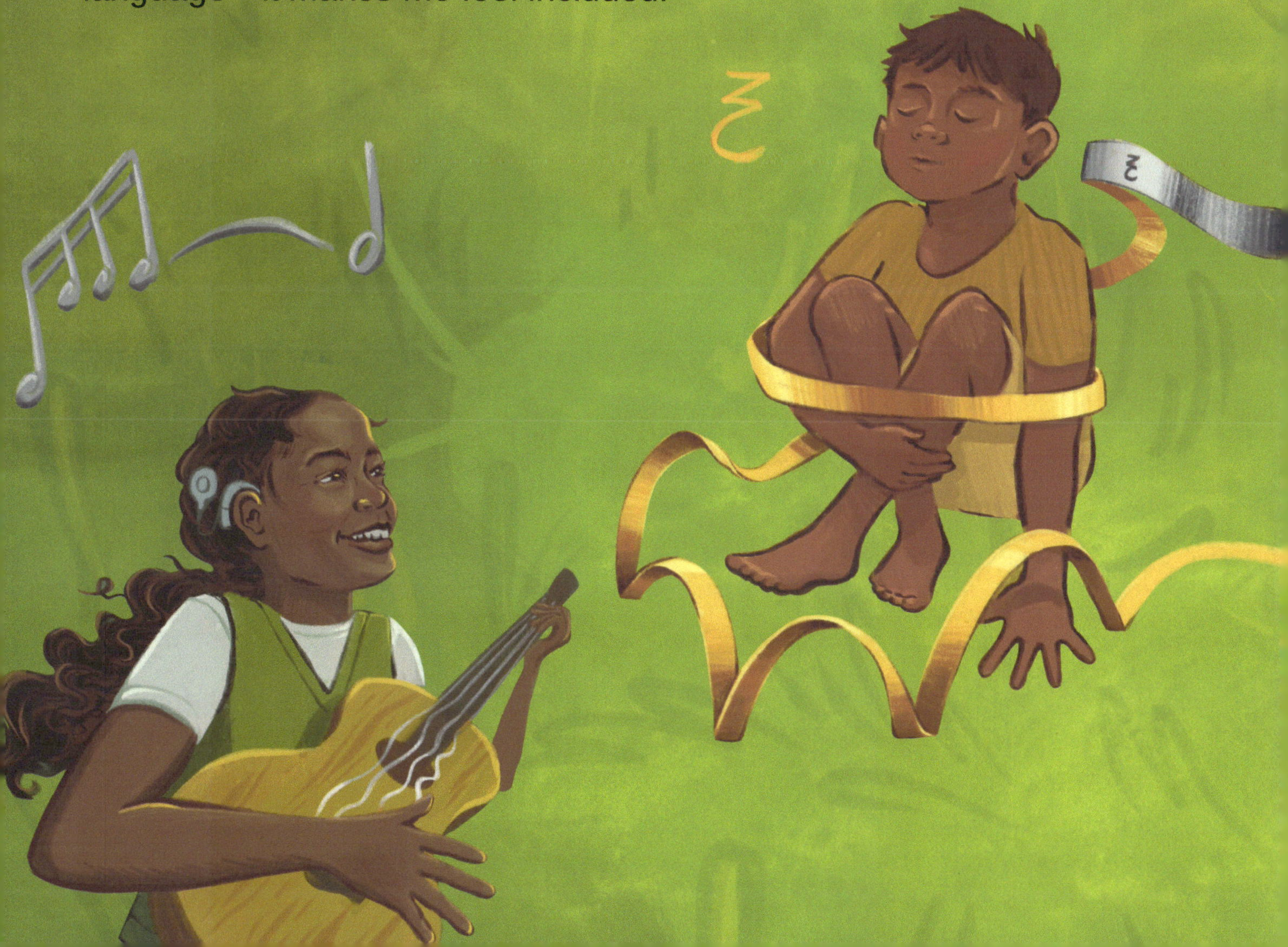

MUSCULAR DYSTROPHY

Green

Muscular dystrophy is a genetic condition where the muscles in the body become weak. The two most common types of muscular dystrophies are Duchenne Muscular Dystrophy and Becker Muscular Dystrophy.

Both conditions have a defective gene on the X chromosome. The X chromosome is one of two sex chromosomes in a human being. In most females, there are two X chromosomes (XX) and most males have one X and one Y (XY).

In Duchenne and Becker, the genetic abnormality on the X chromosome impairs a protein called dystrophin that is primarily found in muscle cells. The primary symptom of those diagnosed is muscle weakness, especially targeting the legs and feet before the arms and hands. As a result, children have a difficult time walking, running, climbing, and breathing as muscles in the body deteriorate. Diagnosis is often confirmed by a muscle biopsy and genetic testing.

Treatment involves the usage of medications called Glucocorticoids. These treatments help to slow the progression of the disease. Working with rehabilitation specialists to support muscle strengthening and adaptive techniques also improves quality of life.

A Specialist often involved in your care: **Pediatric Neurologist**

Patient Perspective:

Ben

What is something other kids should understand about your condition?

Ben: I can do almost everything other kids can, I just may need to do them a little differently, depending on the situation. I am grateful to participate to the extent I can, but that still doesn't take away the feeling of wanting to still really 'do' the activity.

What helps you feel seen or supported?

Ben: My friends have helped me feel included in sports, even if I can't play. My friends' parents have given me rides to practices, games, and included me at team dinners. Anytime my team has won a championship, they have included me in the trophies or rings they receive.

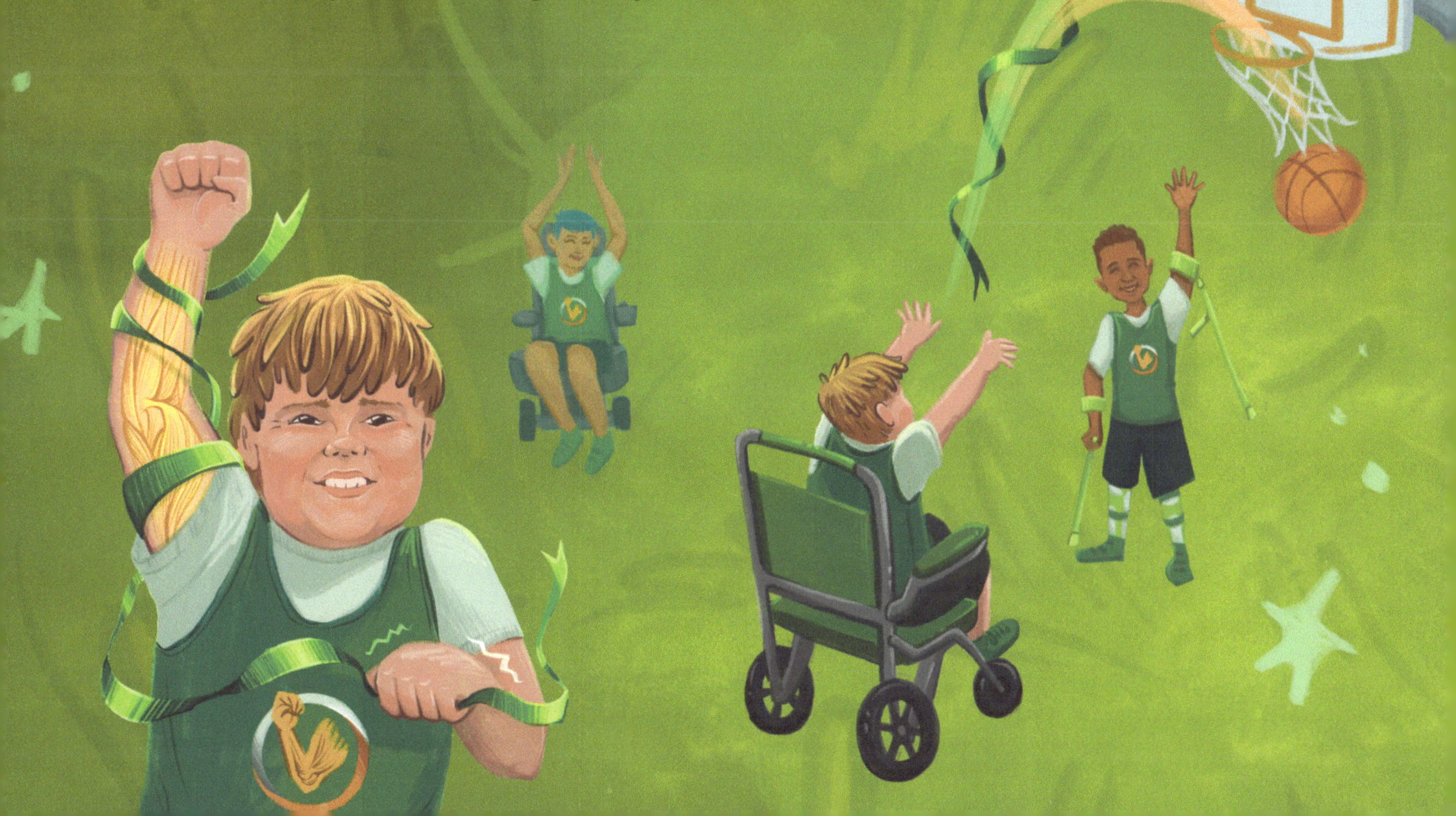

ATTENTION DEFICIT HYPERACTIVITY DISORDER (ADHD)

Orange

ADHD is a common disorder among children and can last into adulthood. Millions of children struggle daily with focusing, controlling impulsive behaviors, or hyperactivity.

Some symptoms are atypical of what society assumes is ADHD, making diagnosis sometimes complicated. Such symptoms may include depression, mood swings, or emotional regulation issues. ADHD may also overlap with other disorders, making specialists all the more valuable when it comes to diagnosis and treatment.

An example of this in the classroom would be having a difficult time not adhering to what is outlined by a teacher, fidgeting, getting out of a seat often, or difficulty staying organized to complete a task at hand.

Children with ADHD may need extra time, encouragement, and grace to help them stay focused, especially since it can have negative impacts as they grow. ADHD has also been studied extensively, and many individuals grow up to be incredibly successful; some call their ADHD their superpower.

A Specialist often involved in your care: **Psychiatrist**

Patient Perspective:

Rowen

What is something other kids should understand about ADHD?

Rowen: I do things differently when I am trying to accomplish a task—school, playing outside, or inside. It's not a bad thing—it just makes your brain a little different. You aren't stupid if you have ADHD, you learn and do things in a different way.

What helps you feel seen or supported?

Rowen: I feel safe when a friend or family member is patient with me. ADHD can be hard to deal with alone; when you have friends and family who give you that extra time and space to be who you are, it makes you feel like you can accomplish anything.

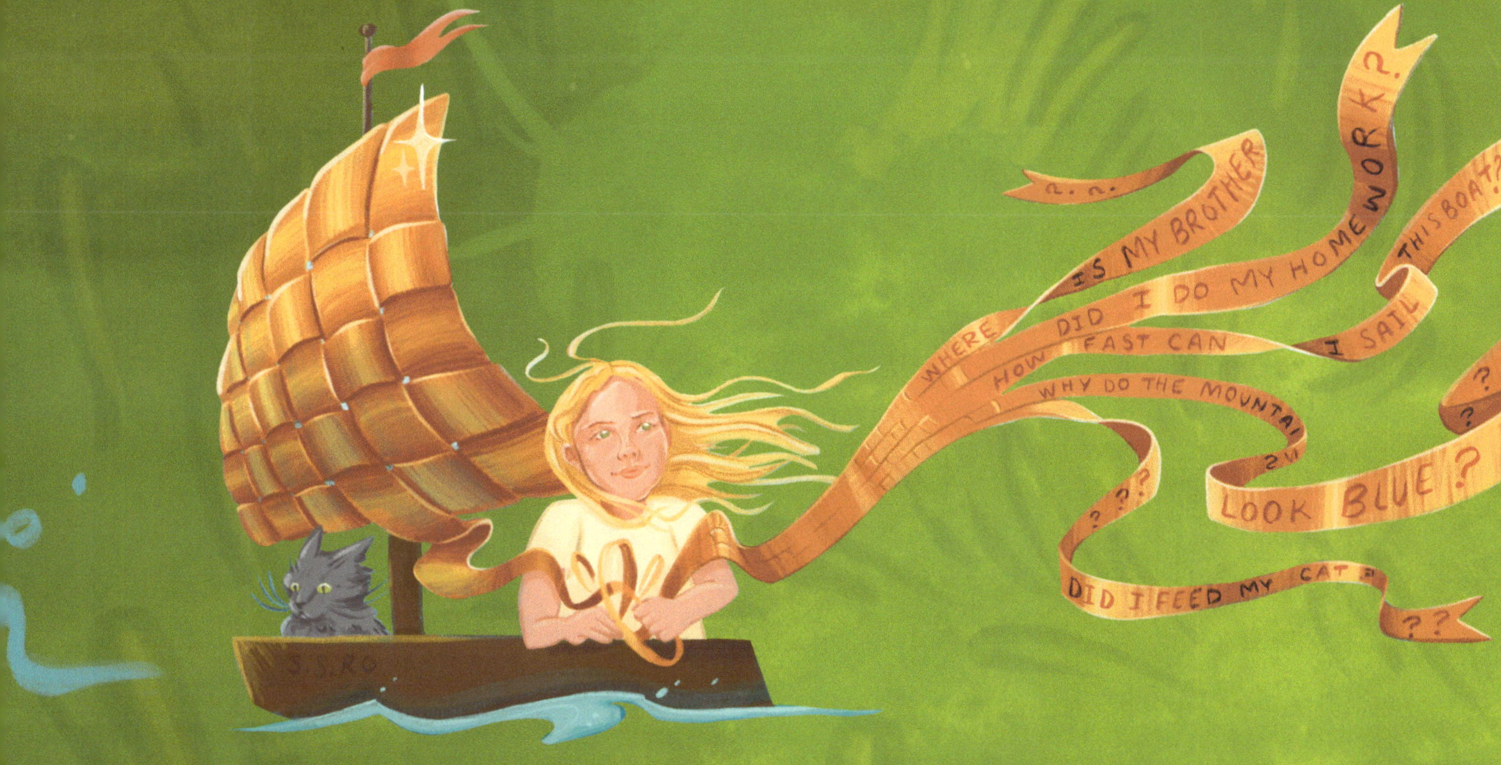
WHERE IS MY BROTHER
DID I DO MY HOMEWORK?
HOW FAST CAN I SAIL THIS BOAT?
WHY DO THE MOUNTAI
LOOK BLUE?
DID I FEED MY CAT
??

DYSLEXIA

Red

Dyslexia is a phonological deficit that is neurologic in origin. It hinders a person's ability to manipulate, decode, and recognize words and language fluently. It occurs in one out of five people, but to varying degrees—sometimes unrecognizable.

Dyslexia may present as a difficulty comprehending, spelling, or deciphering words promptly. Most individuals use the left hemisphere of the brain to process language, whereas those with dyslexia tend to be more right hemisphere dominant. This results in increased time to read and manipulate the written language.

There are standardized tests that can better assess access decoding, fluency, and comprehension to determine if Dyslexia is present, but there is no universal test. Those with Dyslexia can improve word recognition and fluency with the help of adaptive techniques and instruction.

Addressing dyslexia early is the most important step a parent or educator can take. Reading out loud to your child is a great intervention that many experts recommend. In addition, structured literacy programs, multisensory learning techniques, audiobooks and consistent, targeted interventions help build confidence and progress for a child with dyslexia.

A Specialist often involved in your care:
Learning Disability Specialist

Patient Perspective:

Lennon

What is something other kids should understand about Dyslexia?

Lennon: Dyslexia isn't just knowing your left and right. It's more than just flip-flopping a number or letter. Dyslexia is much more; sometimes I can't even explain it myself. But I don't tell people I have Dyslexia because they really won't understand. I am intelligent, I just have to learn things in a much different way.

What helps you feel seen or supported?

Lennon: I feel seen or supported when I am not treated differently or when I am not made fun of because of my dyslexia.

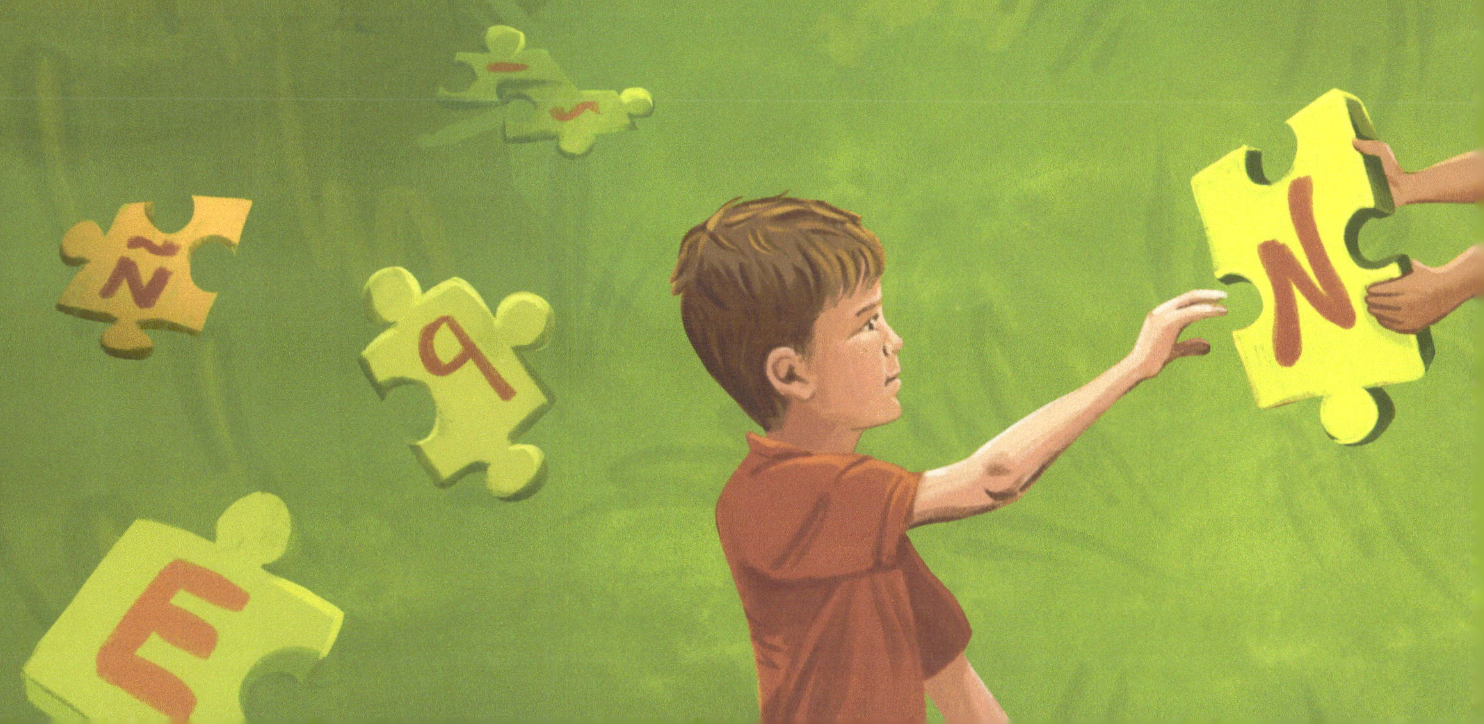

JUVENILE DIABETES

Gray & Blue

An endocrine condition in which the body is unable to properly remove sugar from the bloodstream and store it inside the cells as a form of energy. The endocrine system releases chemical hormones into the bloodstream to carry messages and exert specific tasks all over the body.

Insulin is responsible for regulating blood sugar by storing sugar inside the cells in the form of energy. Sugar comes from the intake of food and drink. When this complex pathway is impaired, it leads to uncontrolled blood sugars. Which is what happens to someone with diabetes.

In Juvenile Diabetes, disruptions of insulin lead to rising levels of blood sugar, which results in fatigue, increased urination, and thirst—often requiring urgent hospitalization.

The diagnosis of Diabetes is made through bloodwork.

Treatment can involve taking medications either by mouth or injections that help regulate the body's blood sugar. Children with diabetes have to monitor their blood sugar levels frequently and be aware of what foods or drinks they consume. Blood sugar can be randomly monitored by pricking the end of a finger or using a continuous glucose monitor (CGM).

A Specialist often involved in your care: **Endocrinologist**

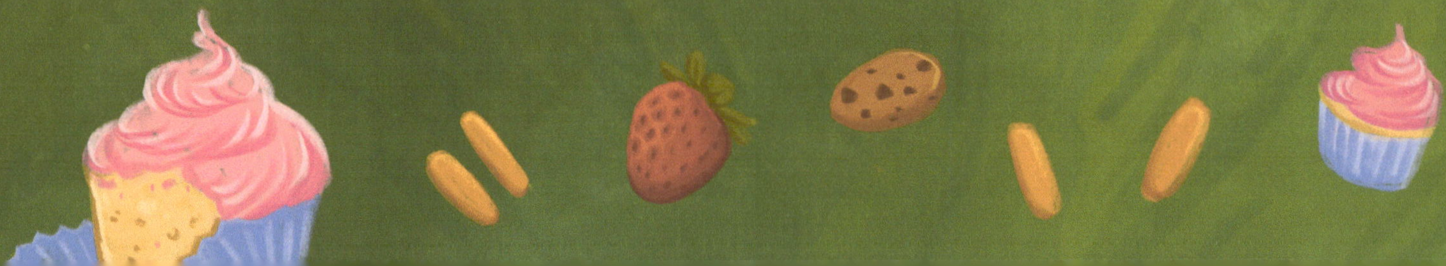

Patient Perspective:

Elliot

What is something other kids should understand about your condition?

Elliot: Diabetes is not as scary as it used to be. Once we knew the diagnosis, we were able to learn about the condition and have a better understanding. The more we understood about diabetes, the more control we felt in managing it.

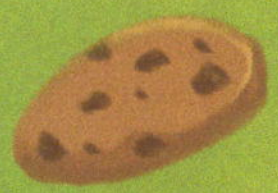

What helps you feel seen or supported?

Elliot: The Juvenile Diabetes Research Foundation (JDRF) walk, friends, and family have helped me feel the most supported. We were recognized as Family of the Year in 2019 by JDRF which made my family and I feel a profound sense of belonging and support.

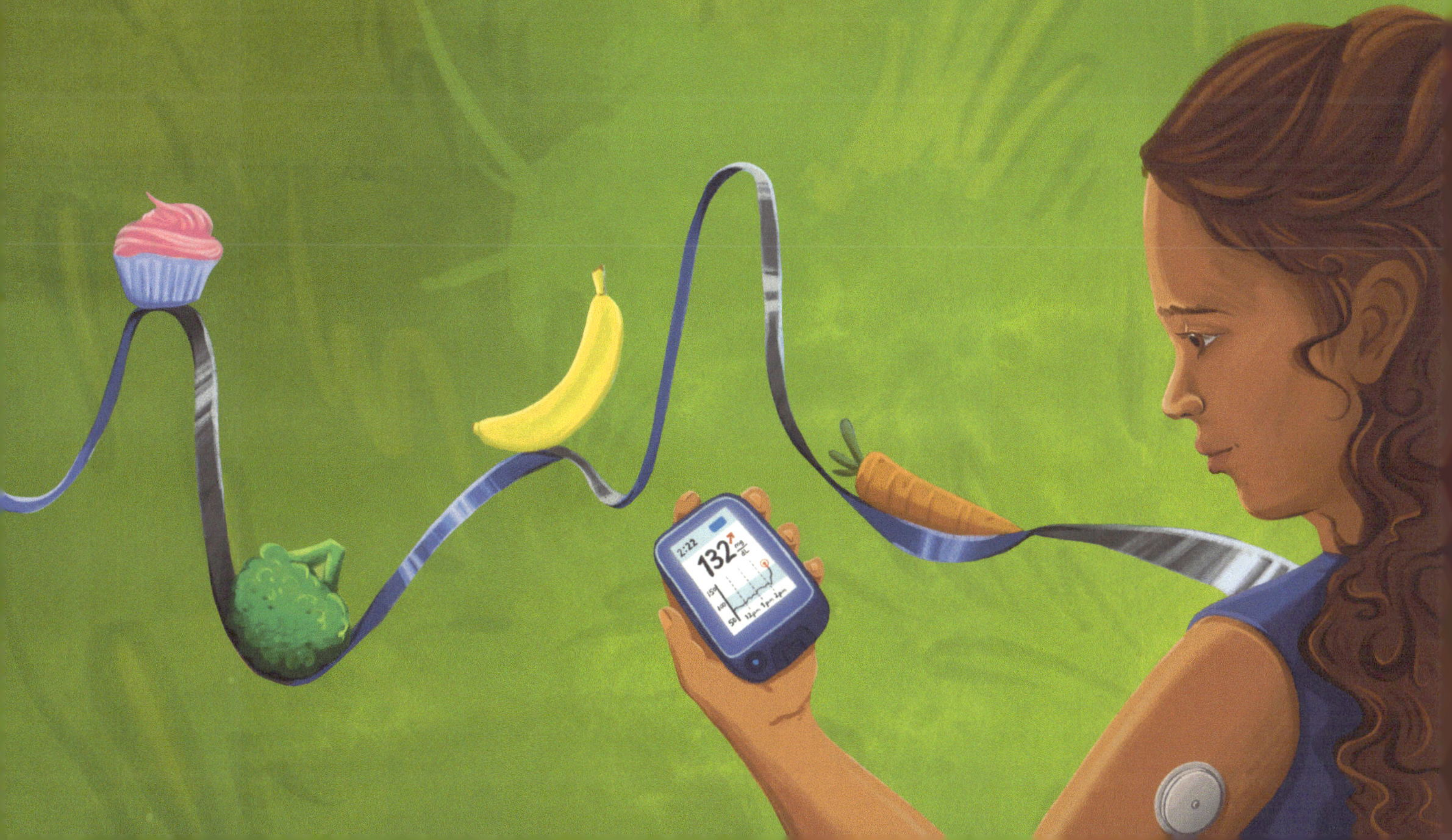

EPILEPSY

Purple

Epilepsy is a neurological disorder of the brain that sends involuntary signals to the body. An epileptic event is often referred to as an unpredictable 'storm' in an individual's brain. As a result, children can experience decreased awareness, loss of consciousness, shaking, jerking, or staring spells.

Seizures are thought to be caused by genetic, structural, metabolic, immune, infectious, or unknown etiologies. Seizures are often diagnosed based on a detailed history, but can be supported by electroencephalography (EEG) or magnetic resonance imaging (MRI). An EEG looks at brain waves and may or may not capture epileptic activity or post-seizure characteristics.

An MRI is an advanced imaging technique to look at the detailed structure of the brain. A multitude of treatment options exist based on the type of seizure, severity, frequency, individual factors, and risk profile.

Medications may be started to help reduce seizure severity and frequency, but often come with a cost due to side effects. Medications may not be effective at stopping the seizures.

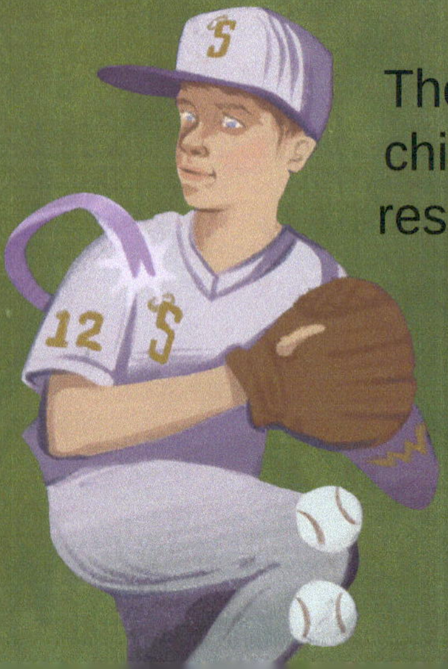

The unpredictable nature results in safety concerns for children who can fall, drown, or sustain other injuries resulting from loss of consciousness.

A Specialist often involved in your care: **Neurologist**

Patient Perspective:

James, Kort and Irelyn

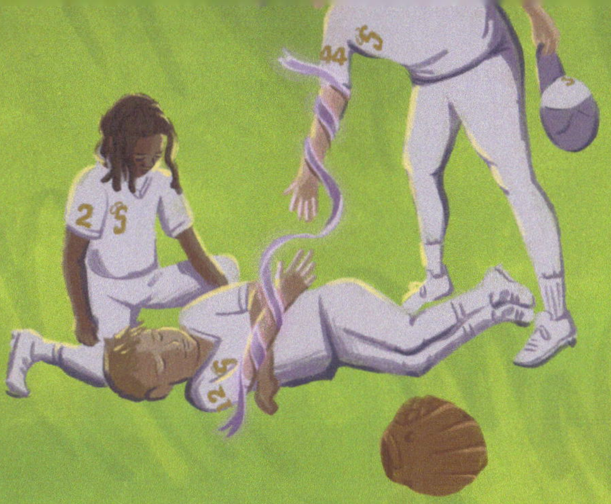

What is something other kids should understand about Epilepsy?

James: Epilepsy is more than just someone dropping to the ground and shaking. There are so many forms of Epilepsy that many people aren't as familiar with. Epilepsy is also remembering to take your medication on time. It is important to get a lot of sleep and make smart choices, so I can stay safe. The scariest part is the unknown of Epilepsy because you never know when a seizure will happen.

What helps you feel seen or supported?

James: The first time I felt seen and supported was when my entire baseball team, The Saints, showed up after my third seizure with purple ribbons on their baseball hats. My family and I were really grateful for that community—even though it was a scary time. I also feel support from my school nurse, teachers, coaches, teammates, and friends who have been trained to help me if I have a seizure.

Irelyn: When people are around me and I get a wobbly arm or feel like a seizure is coming, I feel less scared because they are there to help me.

Kort: I have been supported in a variety of ways like fundraisers, my family and friends who supported me while I was on the Keto diet and those who took time to learn about epilepsy. They were able to understand how hard it can be and ways to help me.

MOBILITY DISORDERS

Silver

There are several disabilities that prevent children from being as mobile as others. Conditions may be temporary or permanent. Mobility may be impaired due to an orthopedic injury, children born without a limb, health ailment, certain illness or accident. A wheelchair, walker, crutches, brace or prosthetics may provide mobility for children to stay active. Oftentimes, children who cannot independently move as well can feel isolated, alone and left out.

Many organizations have brought awareness and opportunity for mobility challenges. Initiatives on accessible and inclusive playgrounds have helped to provide universally designed playgrounds for all to enjoy. Continued growth of paralympics has allowed improved access to activities for those with mobility impairments and highlights their skills and achievements.

A Specialist often involved in your care:

Pediatric - Physical Medicine and Rehabilitation

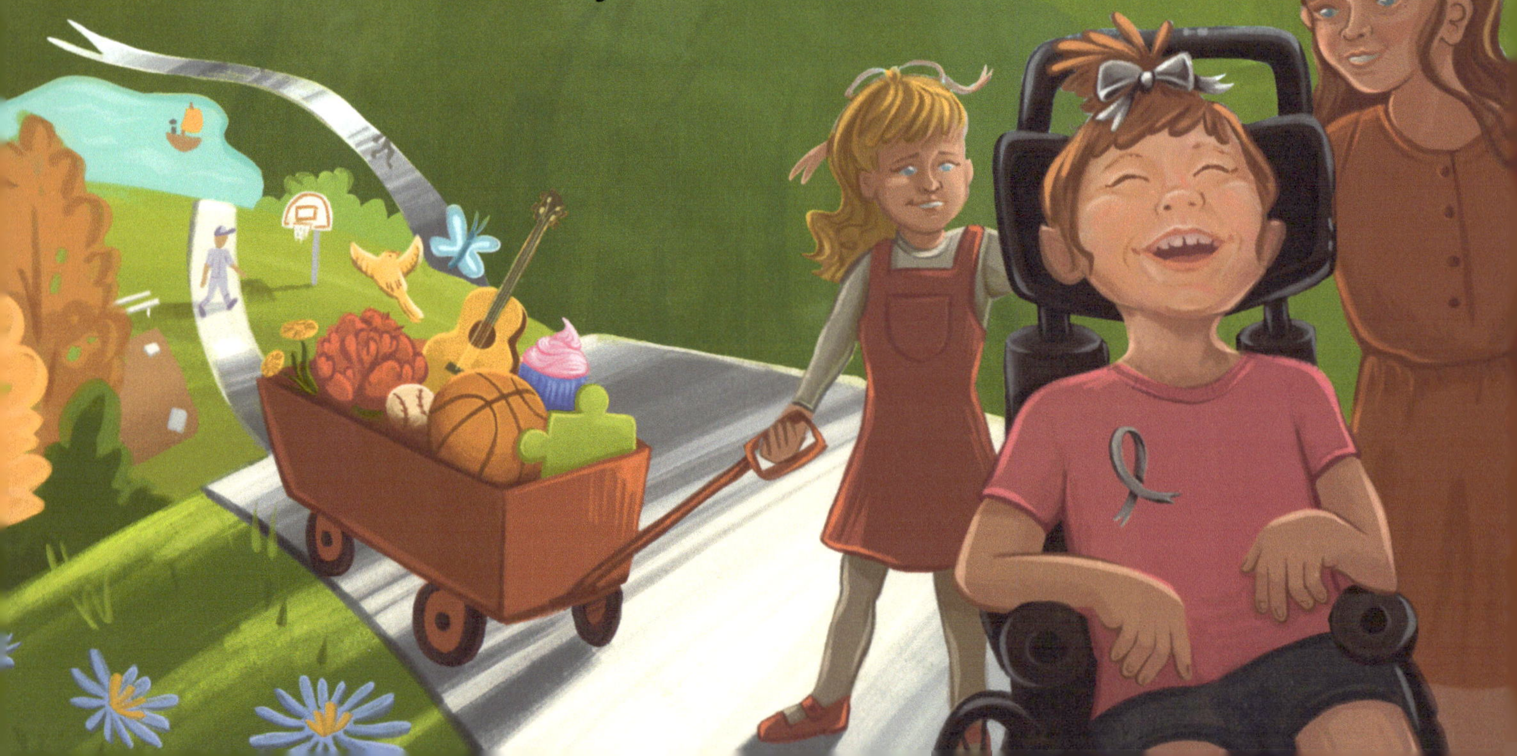

Patient Perspective:

Hazel
(answered by her mother, Emily)

What is something other kids should understand aboutyour condition?

Emily (Hazel): She is still a kid. She loves to be held. She loves books. She loves Mickey Mouse. She is a very simple kid. She wants what any other kid wants. She still has 'enough mind' that she wants those basic things that her sisters want.

What helps you feel seen or supported?

Emily (Hazel): She loves people talking to her! She loves being addressed by name and being included. She loves a "hello." She just wants to listen, take it all in—be present and a part of any group.

ALOPECIA

Light Blue

Alopecia is a hair loss disorder that affects 1 in 1,000 children. Some children can experience smooth patches of missing hair. Others experience complete hair loss on their body.

This disorder can be a result of a child's immune system accidentally attacking their own hair follicles. Alopecia may also occur following a viral illness, exposure to new medication, or from stress.

Alopecia is often seen in other family members or relatives. It can often travel with other systemic disorders such as hypothyroidism, allergies or atopic conditions, vitiligo, or Down Syndrome. Alopecia has variable courses which include resolving spontaneously, progressing further, becoming permanent, or resolving but recurring later.

A history and physical are sufficient for a clinical diagnosis; a scalp biopsy may be obtained to assist in diagnosis.

There are a multitude of treatment options, such as topical ointments, systemic medications, and intralesional injections, with varying degrees of effectiveness. However, the most important treatment needs to focus on psycho-social support as children can suffer from bullying or ostracization.

A Specialist often involved in your care: **Dermatologist**

Patient Perspective:

Michael and Ray

What is something other kids should understand about Alopecia?

Michael: I feel like other kids don't know that Alopecia isn't contagious. A lot of the time, they think it can be passed from one person to the other, but it can't.

Ray: Alopecia doesn't hurt. It doesn't draw me back from achieving my goals. It is visual. Since my diagnosis, people have and continue to stare at me. For me, adults have been worse than kids. Kids will just try to figure out why I have a bald head. I am confident in how I see myself, not what others see from an outward appearance.

What helps you feel seen or supported?

Michael: My mom always takes me to doctor appointments. My friends accept me and know that this is who I am. My mom and dad helped me feel better throughout the bullying. They helped me know how to respond to people. By having my parents support me and talk through my feelings, I know I am supported.

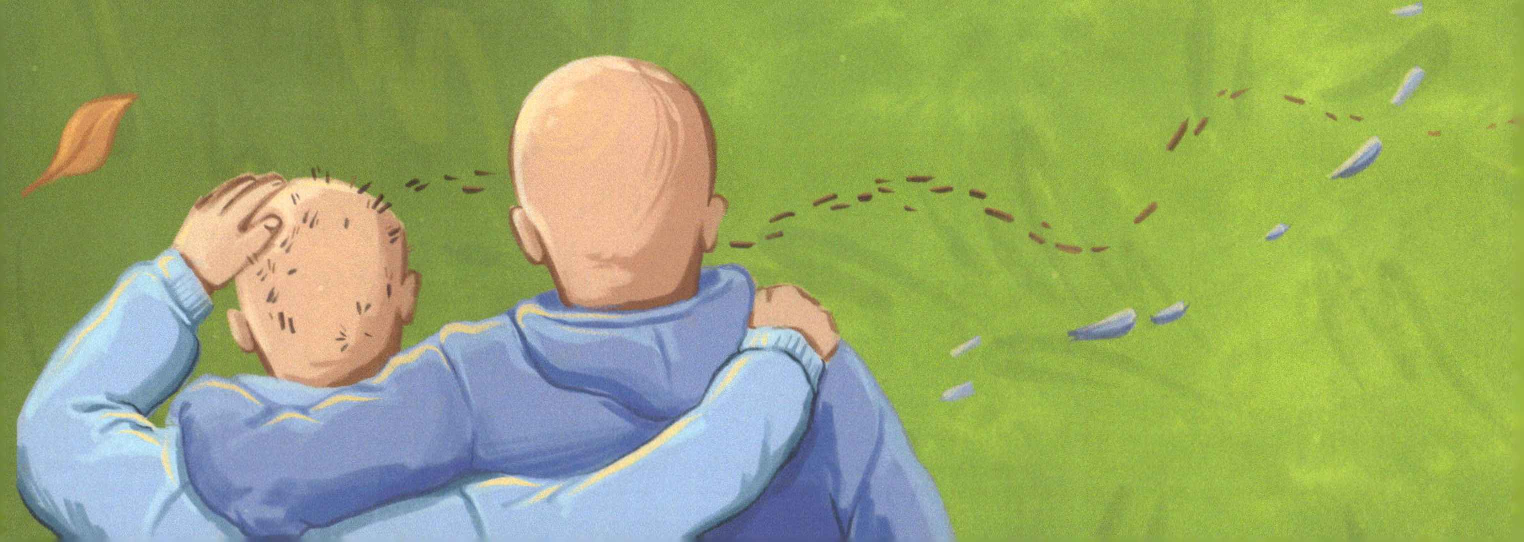

CAREGIVER

Dark Purple

A caregiver is a family member or friend who serves as their loved one's biggest advocate. They often take on nursing, therapeutic, and emotional support roles for their loved one in need.

Depending on the health condition, the caregiver can endure professional pressures, money worries, and fatigue while trying to cope and care for their loved one.

Opportunities arise for us to recognize and offer additional support to caregivers, if we can, with meal trains, childcare for siblings, carpooling, or by simply being present for them so they know they are not alone.

There are also numerous caregiver grants, organizations, government funds, and more available to support these amazing individuals in their efforts to care for those they love.

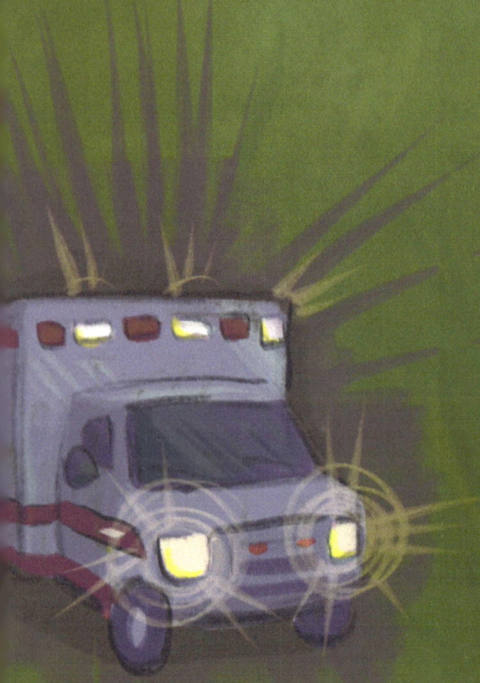

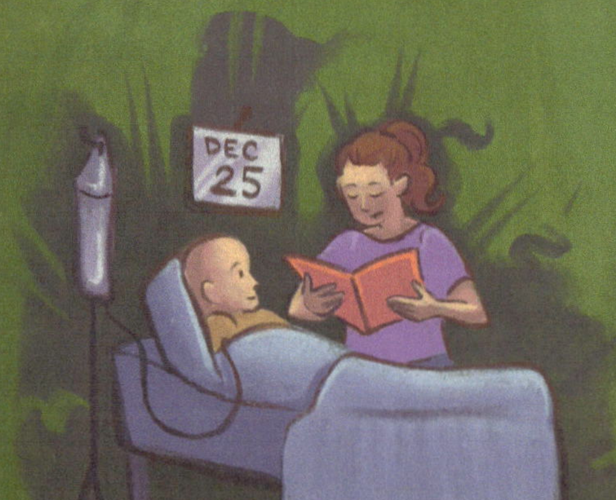

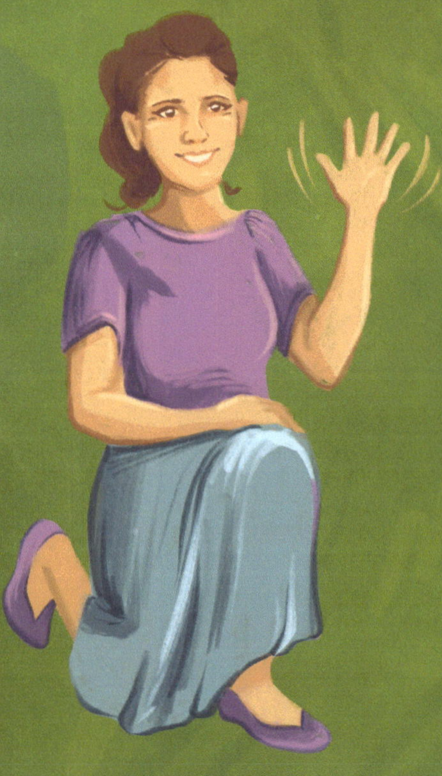

Patient Perspective:

Emily and Kaitlin

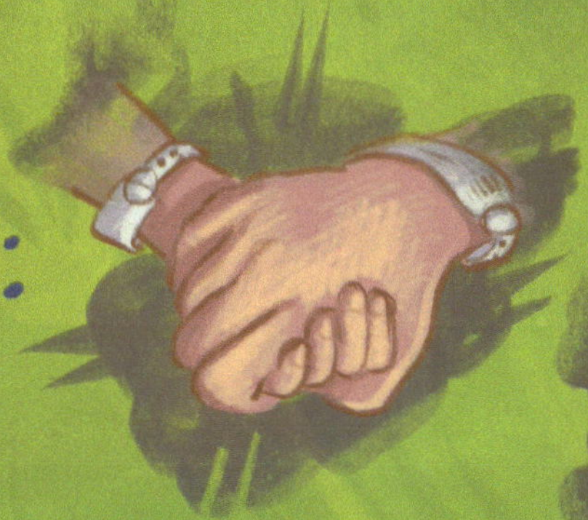

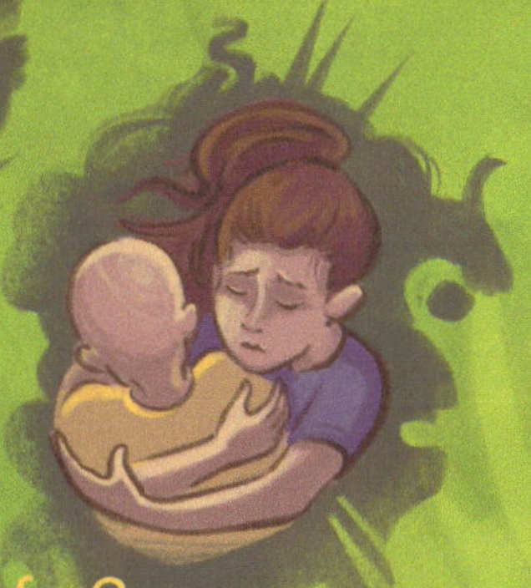

How have these diagnoses affected your life?

Kaitlin: It has touched nearly every aspect of our lives. But through it, our family has learned that there is always another choice. Life is messy, but we still get to decide what we hold onto. As a caregiver, I trust—but verify—and lead with compassion.

What helps you feel seen or supported?

Emily: When others help care for my other children, it relieves guilt from not providing a 'typical' childhood. It is entirely life-giving when friends come to our home and are willing to learn how my child's equipment works, to understand her communication attempts, to provide tangible support, and mostly to not shy away from us, assuming we are too busy or burdened for friendship.

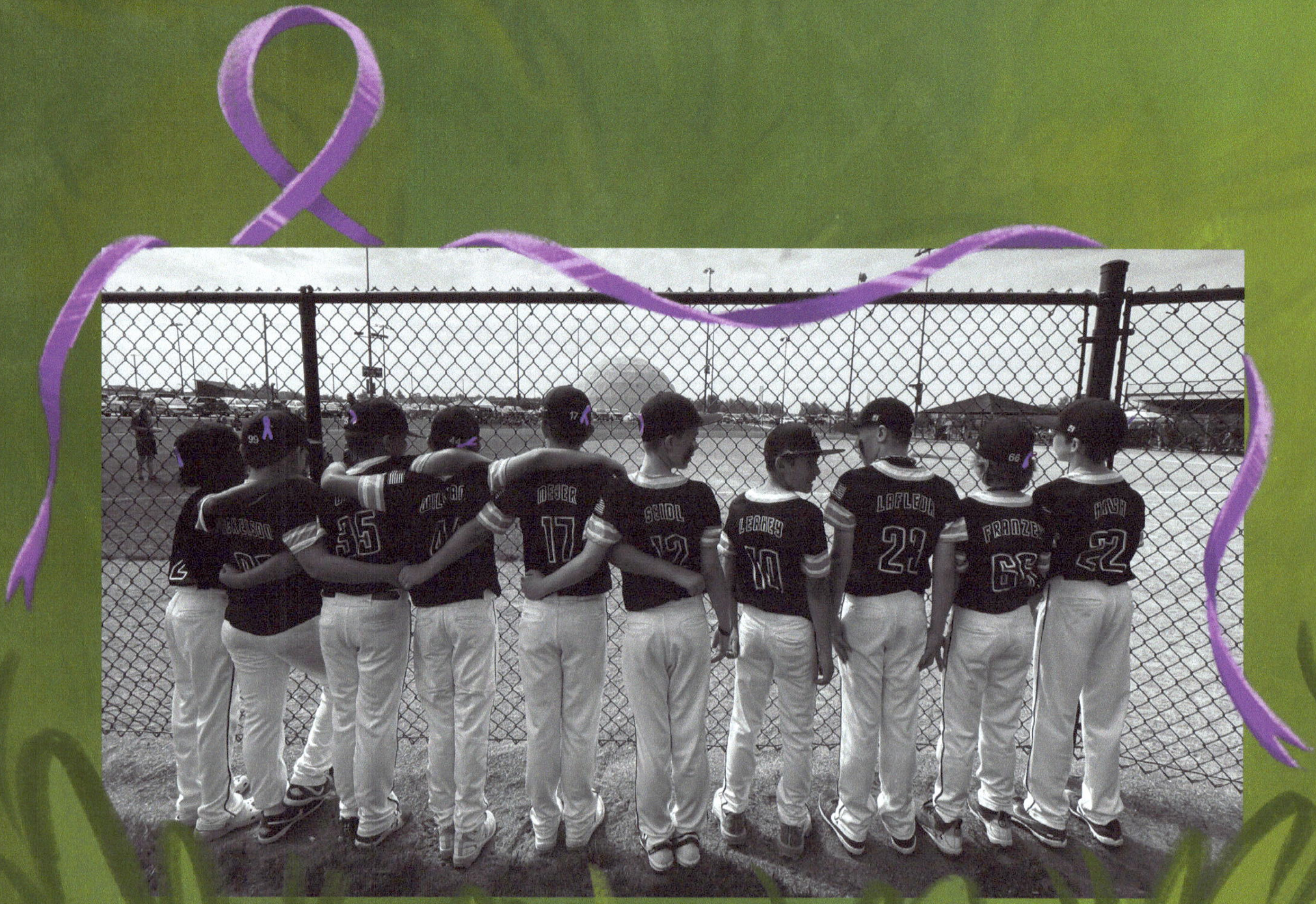

The concept of *The Ribbon* was written in the aftermath of my son James's third grand mal seizure. After three days in the PICU, he was finally discharged. That same weekend, his baseball team was playing in a tournament, and he begged to attend despite his ongoing recovery. Upon arriving at the field, he was greeted by something unexpected: his teammates were all wearing purple ribbons on their hats. In that moment, it became clear that James was not alone; this quiet gesture grew into a powerful symbol and a new story.

(Post tournament)

"Why didn't you tell me I had cancer?" he asked.

"Cancer?" we replied in shock. "You don't have cancer. You have epilepsy."

His voice trembled with disbelief. "But the purple ribbons on my teammates' hats—doesn't that mean I have cancer?"

We immediately wrapped him in our arms. "No," we said gently. "The purple ribbon represents epilepsy awareness. Many medical conditions have a designated color to show support. Your teammates were wearing them to support you."

Later that evening, the concept for *The Ribbon* was formed. What began as a misunderstanding became a tangible symbol of hope. *The Ribbon* exists so that every child knows they are not alone, and that even a single thread can carry immense strength, awareness, and love.

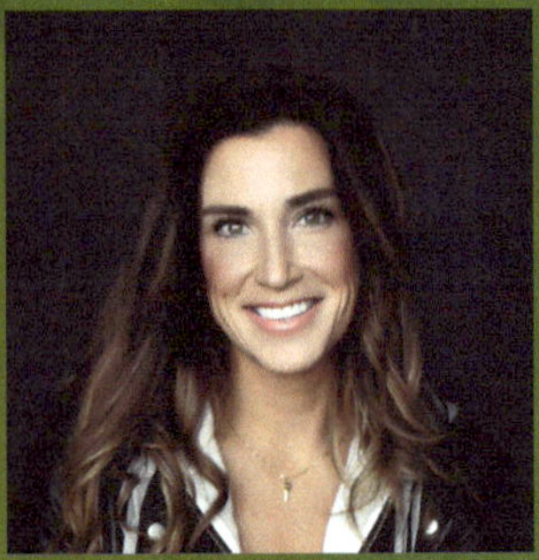

Beth Seidl

Beth Seidl grew up in Iowa, where her love of storytelling and reading took root. She was deeply influenced by her grandfather, Dr. Jim Karabatsos, an English professor at Creighton University; her dynamic and poetic middle school English teacher; and her mother, whose tireless editing continues to shape her work. Her debut children's book, *The Ribbon,* was written for children and families navigating a medical diagnosis, with the hope of fostering unity and representation.

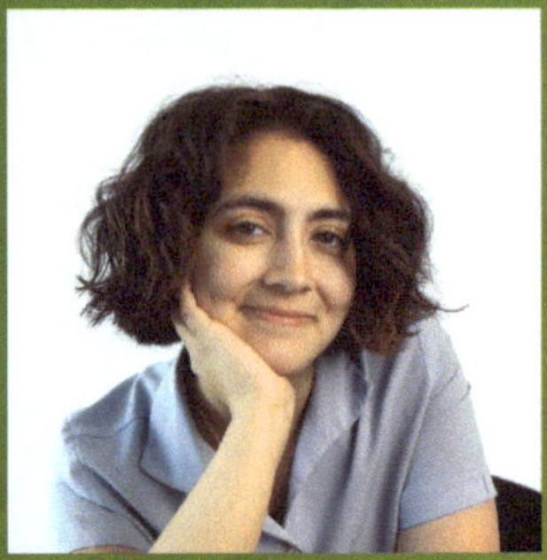

Hannah Roser

Hannah Roser is an Illustrator born in Rochester, NY where she attended Rochester Institute of Technology to study illustration. Hannah currently resides in Southern Pines, NC where she works closely with local businesses in and around Moore County. Her creative design work, editorial illustration and narrative artworks have been featured in serval collaborative projects and art initiatives. Hannah aims to create playful worlds, that are fully saturated with color. When Hannah isn't doodling on her iPad, you can find her walking her dogs, taking a yoga class or sketching in a hammock beneath the pine trees.

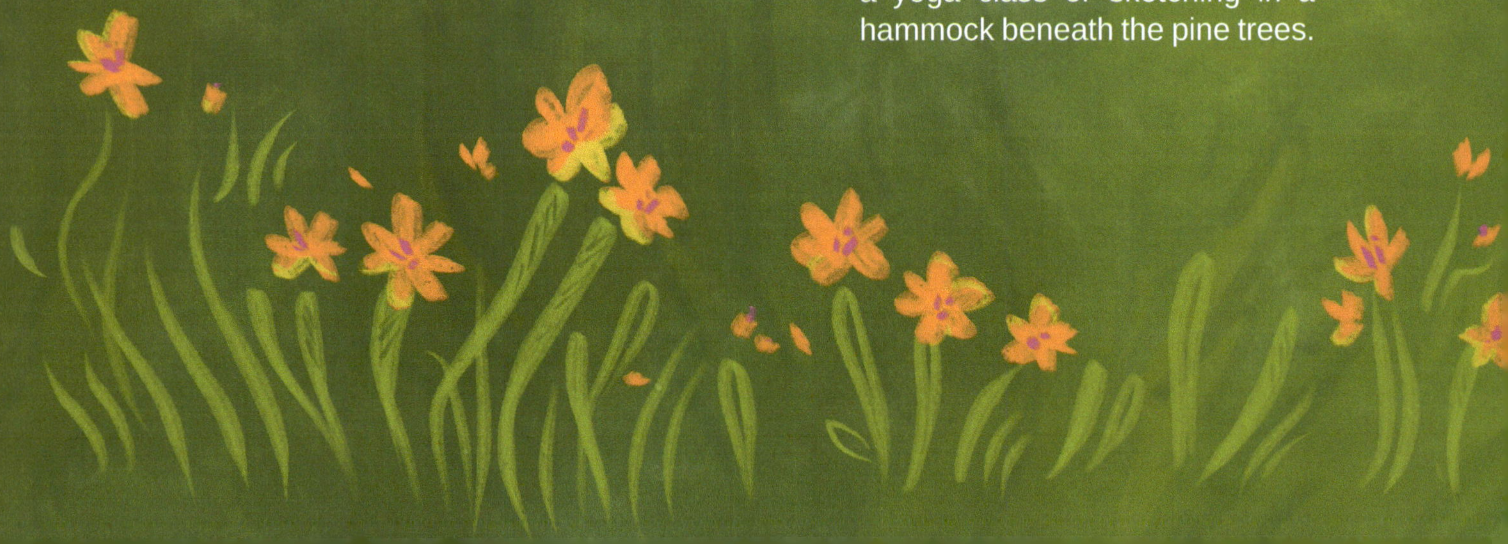

www.ingramcontent.com/pod-product-compliance
Lightning Source LLC
Chambersburg PA
CBHW040302220926
51902CB00031B/117
* 9 7 8 1 9 6 2 3 3 0 0 3 9 *